COLOUR

Gastroenterology and Liver Disease

Peter C. Hayes MD PhD FRCP (Edin)
Senior Lecturer in Medicine
Department of Medicine and Centre for Liver and
Digestive Disorders
Royal Infirmary
Edinburgh

Kenneth J. Simpson MD MRCP
Lecturer in Medicine
Department of Medicine and Centre for Liver and
Digestive Disorders
Royal Infirmary
Edinburgh

Churchill Livingstone

EDINBURGH LONDON MADRID MELBOURNE NEW YORK AND TOKYO 1995

CHURCHILL LIVINGSTONE
Medical Division of Pearson Professional Ltd

Distributed in the United States of America by Churchill
Livingstone Inc., 650 Avenue of the Americas,
New York, N.Y. 10011, and by associated companies,
branches and representatives throughout the world.

First published 1995

ISBN 0-443-04955-6

British Library of Cataloguing in Publication Data
A Catalogue record for this book is available from the
British Library.

Library of Congress Cataloging in Publication Data
A Catalog record for this book is available from the
Library of Congress

For Churchill Livingstone

Publisher
Laurence Hunter
Project Editor
Jim Killgore
Production
Nancy Arnott
Design Direction
Judith Wright
Sales Promotion Executive
Marion Pollock

Printed in Hong Kong
GC/01

Preface

The aim of this book is to provide an illustrated guide to gastroenterology for clinical undergraduates and junior medical staff. We have sought on the whole to avoid the grosser examples of pathology and to keep the illustrations typical of those found in common practice. As well as clinical signs, radiological and endoscopic examples are included since, although they may not be commonly encountered by students, they serve to illustrate the subject under discussion. These pictures we hope will also be valuable to both trainee gastroenterologists and for candidates studying for postgraduate examinations. The text is not aimed to substitute for a text book, but provides, we hope, a succinct and accurate account of the conditions illustrated.

We are very much indebted to many colleagues who have provided illustrations for this book and without whose assistance it could not have been written. We would like to thank Dr R. Thomas and Dr D. Harvey for the use of Figure 66 from *Colour Guide—Paediatrics*, and Dr J.P. Ackers for the use of Figure 63. We would also particularly like to acknowledge the assistance of Drs Niall Finlayson, Doris Redhead, Hugh Gilmour, Juan Piris and Ian Hamilton.

Edinburgh   P.C.H.
1995   K.J.S.

Contents

1 / **Hands**

Examination of the hands is an essential part of all clinical examinations, particularly in a patient with gastro-enterological or hepatic disorders.

Palmar erythema

Erythema of the palms of the hands, particularly in the region of the hypothenar eminence, is a characteristic feature of cirrhosis, particularly of alcoholic aetiology (Fig. 1). The erythema, which is typically blotchy, is also seen in thyrotoxicosis, pregnancy, rheumatoid arthritis and occasionally in healthy subjects.

Dupuytren's contracture

This fibrosis around the flexor tendons is a relatively common abnormality in healthy individuals and may be slightly commoner in patients with cirrhosis and in patients taking phenytoin. It most commonly affects the ring and fifth finger and interferes with manual dexterity (Fig. 2). The cause is unknown but local free radical production generated by the action of xanthine oxidase on hypoxanthine which is found in high concentration in the palmar fascia of these patients has been proposed. For this reason allopurinol may be useful in its management.

Tylosis

Hereditary hyperkeratosis on the palms of the hands and soles of feet. Tylosis is a rare genetic disorder which it is important to recognise, as it is associated with an increased incidence of oesophageal carcinoma.

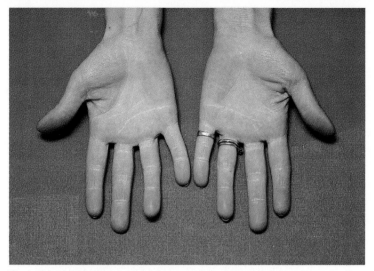

Fig. 1 Palmar erythema.

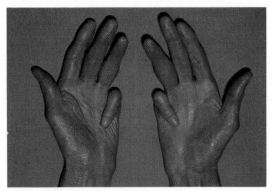

Fig. 2 Dupuytren's contracture.

Scleroderma This condition, most usually the cutaneous manifestation of progressive systemic sclerosis, results in tightening of the skin and is most often identified in the hands and around the mouth. Involvement of the GI tract impairs motility, resulting in dysphagia, impaired gastric emptying and malabsorption.

Finger clubbing This sign is associated with a number of gastrointestinal and liver disorders including cirrhosis, particularly primary biliary cirrhosis or autoimmune chronic active hepatitis, Crohn's disease, ulcerative colitis and coeliac disease. Finger clubbing is an important physical sign and may be an early manifestation of disease and therefore should be sought in all patients. The underlying cause remains unclear but abnormal vascularity and/or platelet dysfunction may be involved. The first stage of clubbing is increased nailbed fluctuation, followed by loss of nailbed angle (Fig. 3), increased curvature of the long axis of the nail and finally soft tissue swelling (Fig. 4). Hypertrophic pulmonary osteo-arthropathy, characterised by tenderness of the wrists or radiological evidence of periosteal elevation and new bone formation, is unusual in gastrointestinal disorders.

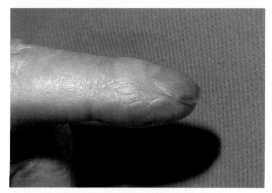

Fig. 3 Loss of nailbed angle.

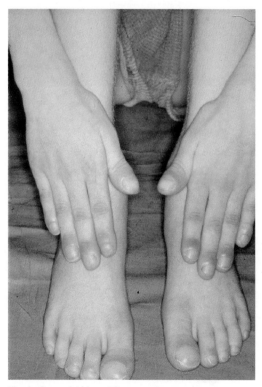

Fig. 4 Gross clubbing of fingers and toes.

2 / **Nails**

Leukonychia This is white discolouration of the nails and is associated with hypoalbuminaemia which occurs, for example, in patients with advanced chronic liver disease (Fig. 5).

Koilonychia Loss of the normal convexity with the nails becoming flat or even concave may be observed, particularly in the elderly. The nails are often thin, ridged and brittle (Fig. 6). At one time the condition was thought to be closely associated with iron deficiency anaemia, but this is now disputed.

Nail dystrophy This may be the result of trauma or fungal infections or be a part of syndromes such as Cronkhite-Canada syndrome, which is characterised by pigmentation, alopecia and intestinal polyps.

Other abnormalities of the nails associated with gastrointestinal disorders include the blueish tint of the lunulae in Wilson's disease, which may also be found in patients abusing phenolphthalein. Polished or shiny nails may be seen in patients with chronic pruritis.

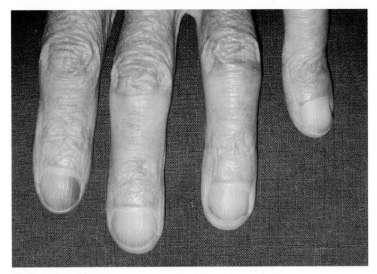

Fig. 5 Leukonychia.

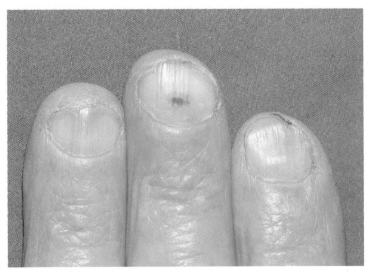

Fig. 6 Koilonychia.

3 / Pigmentation

Anaemia   Anaemia may be detected clinically by pale skin, sometimes with a lemon yellow tinge (e.g. pernicious anaemia), pale mucous membranes and conjunctiva. On the other hand, many patients who are anaemic show no abnormal appearance and others who appear pale are found to have a normal haemoglobin. Causes such as abdominal scars suggestive of gastric surgery should be sought.

Jaundice   This is notoriously difficult to identify particularly in artificial light when mild (Fig. 7). Hyperbilirubinaemia can only be detected reliably once the serum bilirubin exceeds 50 μg/1. The frenulum of the tongue may exhibit a yellow discolouration early on in jaundice. Yellow skin (Fig. 8) with white sclera may be seen in carotenaemia such as occurs in hypothyroidism and vegetarians.

Haemo-
chromatosis   Classically patients with idiopathic haemochromatosis are said to have a slaty-grey complexion, but again the sensitivity and specificity of this sign is poor.

Vitiligo   This may be associated with autoimmune disease such as chronic active hepatitis and pernicious anaemia (Fig. 9).

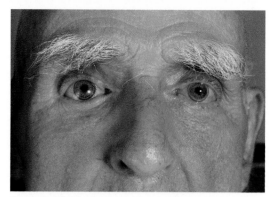

Fig. 7 Jaundiced sclera, note false right eye.

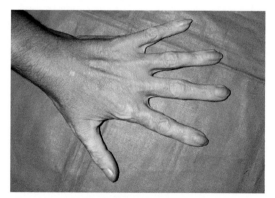

Fig. 8 Jaundiced pigmentation and vitiligo.

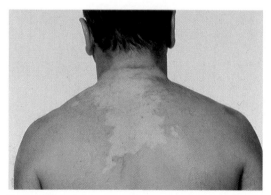

Fig. 9 Vitiligo.

4 / **Skin**

Telangiectasia A classical example of these lesions is seen in patients with hereditary haemorrhagic telangiectasia (Osler-Weber-Rendu syndrome) and in this condition the dilated cutaneous vessels can usually be seen on the lips or tongue (Fig. 10) and are associated with gastrointestinal bleeding. Treatment of such bleeding may be difficult but laser therapy is often effective.

Spider naevi These telangiectatic lesions are not uncommon in normal subjects. The presence of more than three, particularly if they are large, is strongly associated with cirrhosis, particularly of alcoholic aetiology (Fig. 11). They also occur in rheumatoid arthritis, pregnancy and thyrotoxicosis. Their distribution is nearly always in the upper part of the body, i.e. within the drainage region of the superior vena cava and they are particularly common on the face and shoulders. They should be differentiated from Campbell de Morgan spots by their characteristic blanching on pressure and rapid refilling with blood once the pressure is relieved.

Pyoderma gangrenosum These large and often rapidly spreading ulcers with a blue indurated or pustular margin are associated with underlying thrombosis or vasculitis and are seen in patients with ulcerative colitis or Crohn's disease, as well as rheumatoid disease and myeloma (Fig. 12). Treatment is with systemic corticosteroids.

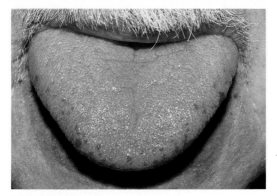

Fig. 10 Telangiectasia on the tongue.

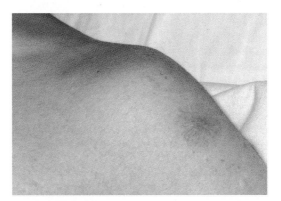

Fig. 11 Spider naevi.

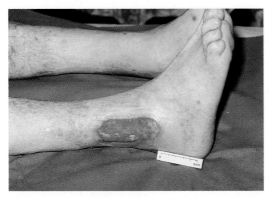

Fig. 12 Pyoderma gangrenosum.

Erythema nodosum

These red raised indurated discrete nodules are most commonly seen on the front of the shins (Fig. 13) and are associated with drug sensitivity (e.g. penicillin, sulphonamides), streptococcal and mycoplasma infections, tuberculosis, sarcoidosis, ulcerative colitis and Crohn's disease. They should be differentiated from cellulitis, phlebitis and trauma. Treatment is primarily symptomatic as the lesion is generally self-limiting.

Porphyria cutanea tarda

This blistering scarring skin disorder (Fig. 14), which affects mainly sun-exposed areas, has long been known to be associated with iron overload secondary to alcoholic liver disease, but more recently there is good evidence to implicate the hepatitis C virus. In many patients venesection produces improvement.

Acanthosis nigricans

This is a condition characterised by a brown or blackish thickened, velvet area of skin commonly in the axilla, on the back of the neck, in the perianal or the inguinal region, which in adults is frequently associated with intra-abdominal malignancy, particularly of the pancreas (Fig. 15).

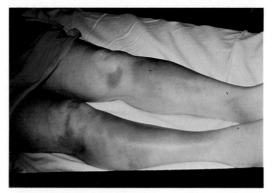

Fig. 13 Erythema nodosum.

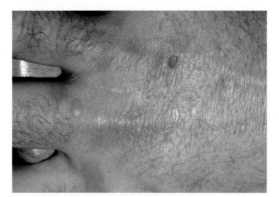

Fig. 14 Skin blisters of porphyria cutanea tarda.

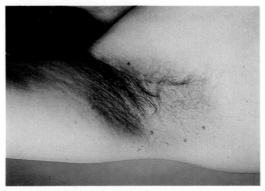

Fig. 15 Acanthosis nigricans.

5 / Face

Peutz-Jegher's syndrome
This is characterised by multiple pigmented lentigines around the lips (Fig. 16), gums and tips of the fingers with an autosomal dominant pattern of inheritance. Clinically the most important aspect of this syndrome is small intestinal polyposis which not uncommonly results in intestinal bleeding.

Carcinoid syndrome
Flushing of the face, neck and upper chest is a characteristic feature of carcinoid syndrome. The swelling may be transient lasting only for hours or may persist for days. Wheezing and diarrhoea are other features. Flushing may be precipitated by alcohol, food or exercise and is due to circulating humoral products of carcinoid tumours, inactivation of which is impaired by hepatic metastases. In such cases hepatomegaly is the usual finding whilst in ovarian and bronchial carcinoids the syndrome may occur without liver metastases.

Xanthelasma
These are wash-leather plaques which occur on both the upper and lower eyelids (Fig. 17). Although these may occur in healthy subjects with normal blood lipids they are commonly seen in patients with hypercholesterolaemia such as may occur with chronic cholestasis (Fig. 18). They are a characteristic feature of primary biliary cirrhosis and may precede the development of jaundice.

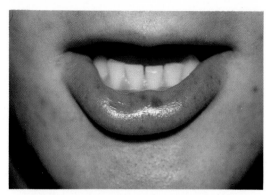

Fig. 16 Pigmented lesions in Peutz-Jegher's syndrome.

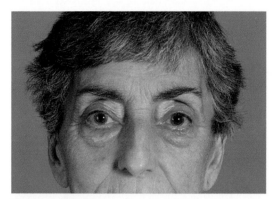

Fig. 17 Xanthelasma.

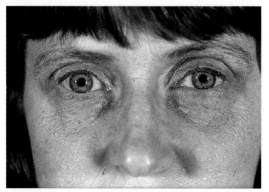

Fig. 18 Xanthelasma and jaundiced sclera in a patient with chronic cholestasis.

Kayser-Fleischer rings	This is a classical feature of Wilson's disease and is caused by condensation of brown copper-containing granules in Descemet's membrane near the limbus of the eye. The eye should be viewed obliquely from above with a magnifying glass and the discolouration is seen at a lower margin of the cornea (Fig. 19). The sign, although characteristic, is not pathognomonic for Wilson's disease and may occasionally be seen in primary biliary cirrhosis and chronic active hepatitis.
Sjögren's syndrome	Abnormal dryness of the eyes may lead to keratitis (keratoconjunctivitis sicca). This results in painful gritty eyes which require treatment with artificial tears. The condition is associated with primary biliary cirrhosis.
Iritis	This is characterised by injection of the circumcorneal blood vessels and may be a manifestation of ulcerative colitis as well as sarcoidosis, ankylosing spondylitis, Reiter's syndrome, rheumatoid disease and toxoplasmosis.
Scleroderma	Tightening of the skin over the nose and around the mouth (Fig. 20) often associated with telangiectases is characteristic of scleroderma.
Parotid enlargement	Parotitis is not uncommonly seen in alcoholic patients, particularly those with alcoholic cirrhosis and is due to a combination of dehydration, malnutrition and sex hormone disturbances. It is also a feature of Sjögren's syndrome.

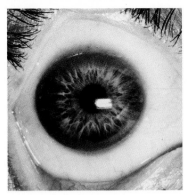

Fig. 19 Kayser-Fleischer ring.

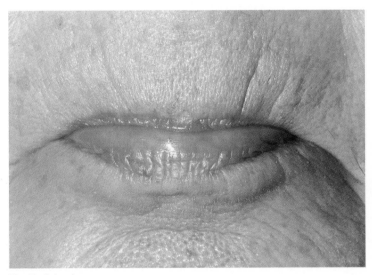

Fig. 20 Scleroderma.

6 / Mouth

Aphthous ulceration   This is a very common condition particularly in adolescents and young adults characterised by crops of vesicles which rupture forming shallow painful ulcers. They usually heal in a few days without scarring and have a very limited significance, although they are occasionally associated with inflammatory bowel disease and coeliac disease. Larger painful ulcers are a feature of Behçet's disease, which presents predominantly in young women, or herpes zoster (Fig. 21). Other features of Behçet's include genital ulcers and recurrent ocular problems including conjunctivitis and recurrent iritis.

Crohn's disease   The inflammatory lesions of Crohn's disease can occur anywhere in the GI tract. Aphthous and linear oral ulcers (Fig. 22) may be a feature, as may involvement of the lips (Fig. 23). This may result in disfiguring thickening which requires corticosteroid treatment.

Glossitis   Atrophic glossitis resulting in a shiny smooth tongue may be caused by malabsorption of iron and vitamin B including B12. In patients with iron deficiency anaemia it may be associated with angular cheilitis. Furring of the tongue is not uncommon in febrile patients and in those with liver and renal failure.

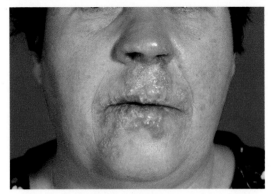

Fig. 21 Oral herpes zoster infection.

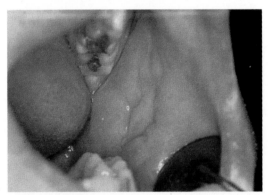

Fig. 22 Oral Crohn's disease.

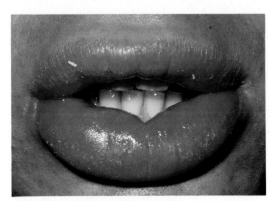

Fig. 23 Crohn's disease affecting the lips.

7 / Pharynx

Candidiasis

Candidiasis of the mouth and pharynx is common (Fig. 24). It is associated with antibiotic and steroid therapy, and poor dental hygiene (e.g. sleeping with dentures in place). It is also seen in immunocompromised patients such as those with AIDS, although it is oesophageal rather than pharyngeal candidiasis which is of diagnostic importance. It is characterised by creamy white patches which cannot be easily scraped away, with underlying inflammation.

Acute pharyngitis

This is most often due to viral infection (e.g. Epstein-Barr virus) or *Streptococcus pyogenes*. Most often the complaint is only of a sore throat, but dysphagia may occur. Signs include pharyngeal inflammation and lymphoid hypertrophy with or without an exudate. Complications include peritonsillar and parapharyngeal abscesses.

Pharyngeal pouch

A pharyngeal diverticulum or Zenker's pouch is thought to be due to a congenital weakness associated with high pressure related to a oesophageal spasm or hyperactive upper oesophageal sphincter. It arises between the oblique fibres of the inferior constrictor and the transverse fibres of the cricopharyngeous. It is commoner in men and results in collection of mucus in the throat followed by dysphagia. Regurgitation, coughing and halitosis are also not uncommon. The diagnosis is usually made by barium swallow (Fig. 25), and the possibility of a pharyngeal pouch should be considered in all patients with dysphagia and when undertaking an upper GI endoscopy, to avoid perforation. The treatment is surgical.

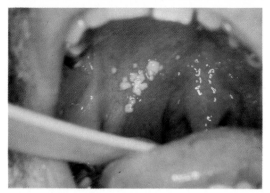

Fig. 24 Oral candidiasis.

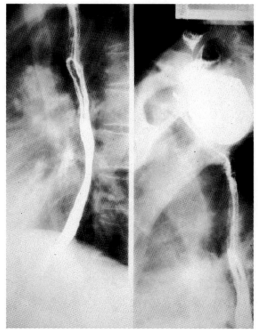

Fig. 25 Barium swallow showing a pharyngeal pouch.

8 / Oesophagus

Fistulae and perforation

The commonest cause of acquired fistulae is malignancy. The connection may be between the oesophagus and the aorta, bronchi or pleural space. Benign fistulae may result from perforation or surgery. The commonest cause of perforation is upper GI endoscopy.

Clinical features
These include, pain and fever, dyspnoea, shock and surgical emphysema (Figs 26 & 27).

Treatment
High instrumental perforations can be treated conservatively with fasting and antibiotics whilst lower perforations require immediate surgical intervention.

Mucosal ring

The mucosal or Schatzki ring lies at the lower end of the oesophagus and is composed of fibrous tissue. Although it is probably developmental it usually produces symptoms after the sixth decade.

Clinical features
Symptoms include episodic dysphagia particularly with meat and sometimes made worse by emotional stress. The diagnosis may be confirmed radiologically or at endoscopy.

Treatment
Treatment is usually symptomatic although pneumatic dilatation may be required.

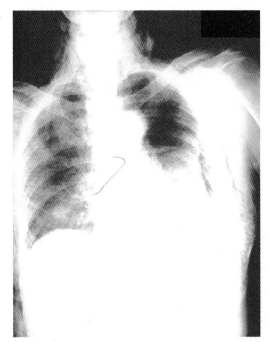

Fig. 26 Chest X-ray following oesophageal perforation showing surgical emphysema and a left-sided pneumothorax.

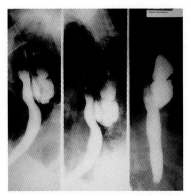

Fig. 27 Oesophageal perforation.

Oesophageal web

Clinical features
In the Paterson-Kelly syndrome a web in the pharynx may develop and cause dysphagia. Other features include iron deficiency anaemia, angular stomatitis, glossitis and achlorhydria.

Diagnosis
Diagnosis is confirmed radiologically (Fig. 28) and endoscopically. This latter is preferable as the condition is associated with an increased risk of cancer. Endoscopy frequently ruptures the connective tissue web before it is visualised and this usually relieves the dysphagia.

Oesophagitis

Aetiology
The commonest cause for oesophagitis is reflux of acid (see below). Other causes though less common should not be forgotten and include reflux of bile and infection. Oesophageal candidiasis may occur in immunosuppressed patients or in those taking antibiotics or in the debilitated (Fig. 29).

Clinical features
Symptoms include painful dysphagia, heartburn and retrosternal chest pain and it should be noted that in candidiasis oral involvement is not always present.

Diagnosis
Diagnosis made endoscopically can be confirmed histologically or by taking brushings. Viral infection of the oesophagus, particularly herpes virus, may occur in debilitated patients. Inflammation and ulceration may also occur due to drugs particularly in those with oesophageal disease, especially if medication is taken without water. Drugs most commonly implicated are tetracycline and Slow K.

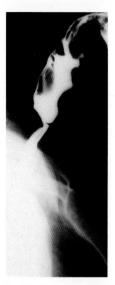

Fig. 28 Upper oesophageal web.

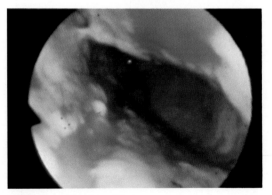

Fig. 29 Oesophageal candidiasis.

Reflux oesophagitis

Aetiology This is common and due to regurgitation of acid through the lower oesophageal sphincter. Underlying causes include incompetence of the lower oesophageal sphincter, impaired motility resulting in reduced acid clearance once regurgitated and it is occasionally due to increased intragastric pressure associated with gastric outlet obstruction, or gastroparesis. Risk factors include obesity, alcohol consumption, pregnancy and cigarette smoking.

Clinical features The condition may be asymptomatic although heartburn and water brash and later dysphagia are characteristic. The diagnosis is made either radiologically or preferably endoscopically. This latter allows grading of oesophagitis from mild (grade I) (Fig. 30) to severe circumferential ulceration (grade IV) (Figs 31 & 32).

Complications Complications include oesophageal stricture, haemorrhage, pulmonary aspiration and Barrett's oesophagus which is associated with an increased risk of oesophageal carcinoma.

Treatment Treatment includes general measures such as weight loss, stopping smoking, reducing alcohol and caffeine intake and elevating the head of the bed at night. Pharmacological treatment includes antacids, H_2 antagonists and omeprazole, mucosal protecting agents such as sucralfate and pro-motility drugs such as cisapride. Omeprazole is particularly effective in healing oesophagitis, but in many cases because of the chronic nature of the underlying cause treatment may have to be prolonged.

Barrett's oesophagus

As mentioned above Barrett's oesophagus, with replacement of oesophageal squamous epithelium by gastric mucosa, is associated with chronic reflux oesophagitis. The transformed mucosa is prone to ulceration from bleeding and is premalignant. Unfortunately once present regression even with optimal treatment is rare.

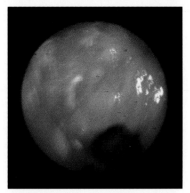

Fig. 30 Mild reflux oesophagitis.

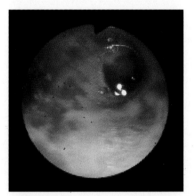

Fig. 31 Haemorrhagic oesophagitis.

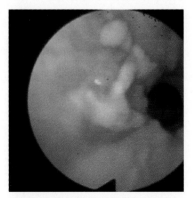

Fig. 32 Oesophageal ulceration due to reflux.

Hiatus hernia

Prevalence The commonest form of hiatus hernia is the sliding variety where the gastro-oesophageal junction migrates from the diaphragmatic hiatus into the chest. This results in disruption of the lower oesophageal sphincter mechanism and predisposes to reflux of gastric acid. Hiatus hernia is extremely common, particularly in those over the age of 40 and its prevalence varies with investigative techniques.

Clinical features Many patients with hiatus hernia do not suffer either from heartburn or reflux oesophagitis and it should be remembered that it is the reflux oesophagitis that is clinically important rather than the presence of a hiatus hernia. Another form is the para-oesophageal hiatus hernia where the gastro-oesophageal junction remains in its normal position and the fundus of the stomach herniates through the oesophageal hiatus anterior to the oesophagus (Fig. 33). In some cases the entire stomach and even other abdominal organs may enter the hernial sac. In these patients, since the lower oesophageal sphincter is competent, reflux is not usual and symptoms include epigastric fullness, dyspepsia, dysphagia and breathlessness after food. Gastric volvulus may occur and result in gangrene of the stomach.

Diagnosis The sliding hiatus hernia is best identified endoscopically. A para-oesophageal hernia may be recognised on a plain chest X-ray where the fluid level is seen behind the heart (Fig. 34) and the diagnosis is best made by barium swallow and meal which shows partial obstruction of the gastro-oesophageal junction and a segment of intrathoracic stomach.

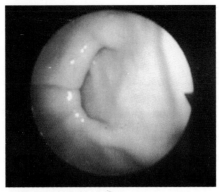

Fig. 33 Para-oesophageal hiatus hernia.

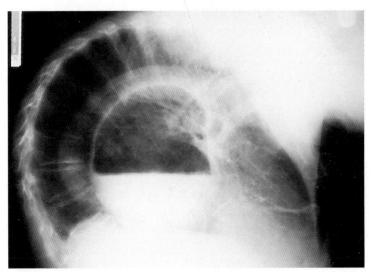

Fig. 34 Chest X-ray showing fluid level in a hiatus hernia.

Strictures

Strictures of the oesophagus are most often benign and are related to acid reflux causing fibrosis. However, oesophageal carcinoma also often presents with stricture formation.

Clinical features
Both present with progressive dysphagia and although weight loss is more characteristic in those with malignancy, it may also be pronounced in those with benign disease.

Diagnosis
Although the diagnosis can be made radiologically (Fig. 35) endoscopy is preferable as it allows histological confirmation as well as dilatation (Fig. 37).

Carcinoma

Oesophageal cancer accounts for approximately 1% of all tumours and arises most frequently in the lower third of the oesophagus. The tumour is commonly of the squamous type, although adenocarcinoma, which may be of gastric origin, may occur in the lower oesophagus.

Risk factors
Risk factors include alcohol abuse and smoking, chronic peptic oesophagitis, Barrett's syndrome, achalasia and radiation exposure.

Clinical features
Patients are usually over the age of 50 and in 85% present with dysphagia although anorexia, weight loss, anaemia and haematemesis are not uncommon.

Diagnosis
The diagnosis may be made by barium swallow (Fig. 36) or, better, by endoscopy which also allows histological confirmation.

Treatment
Unfortunately curative surgery is only an option in a small minority and treatment is usually palliative. Treatment options include surgery, intubation, e.g. the Celestin pulsion tube, radiotherapy, laser forage and ethanol tumour necrosis.

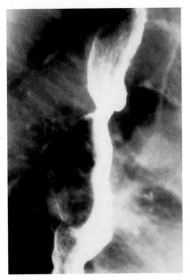

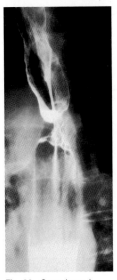

Fig. 35 Peptic oesophageal stricture.

Fig. 36 Oesophageal carcinoma.

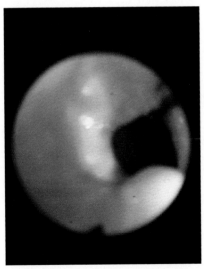

Fig. 37 Oesophageal stricture and ulceration.

Achalasia

The best known motility disorder of the oesophagus is achalasia where an increased resting pressure of the lower oesophageal sphincter and impaired relaxation is characteristic. These abnormalities are due to loss of smooth muscle innervation of the oesophagus in this region. The cause of the abnormality is unknown.

Clinical features

Patients usually present in early middle age with slowly progressive dysphagia for both solids and liquids. Symptoms are often intermittent and may have been present for years, gradually increasing in severity before presentation. Retrosternal chest pain is a prominent symptom in approximately one third of cases.

Diagnosis

Diagnosis is usually made by a combination of barium radiology (Fig. 38) and endoscopy. The former shows dilatation of the proximal oesophagus with a smooth tapered lower end producing the characteristic 'bird's beak' appearance.
Cineradiography may be necessary in less advanced cases and demonstrates failure of primary peristalsis to clear the oesophagus. Upper GI endoscopy is usually undertaken to confirm the absence of malignancy. Manometric studies are valuable in confirming the diagnosis.

Treatment

Treatment may be undertaken using pneumostatic or hydrostatic balloon dilatation (Fig. 39), which often results in symptomatic improvement, but is not without risks of oesophageal perforation. Surgical options include Heller's operation, for which incisions are made on the circular muscle of the gastro-oesophageal junction.

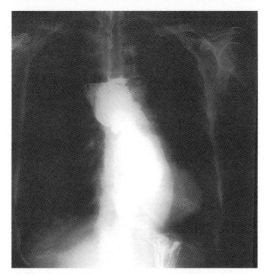

Fig. 38 Barium swallow showing typical changes of achalasia.

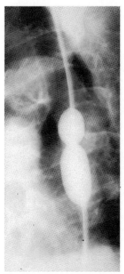

Fig. 39 Pneumatic dilatation of achalasia.

Diffuse oesophageal spasm

Clinical features A second oesophageal dysmotility syndrome is diffuse oesophageal spasm. This condition of unknown cause presents either with dysphagia—which is typically intermittent, non-progressive and is present for both solids and liquids and is often related to ingestion of cold fluids or large boluses of food—or chest pain. This latter may simulate the pain of cardiac ischaemia where a relationship between the pain and swallowing is only found in approximately 50% of cases.

Diagnosis The diagnosis is generally made by barium radiology where the classical appearance of a 'nutcracker' or 'corkscrew' oesophagus may be found (Fig. 40). However, spasm may be intermittent and a normal barium swallow does not exclude the diagnosis. Manometry is the investigation of choice and characteristically shows high amplitude non-pulsatile contractions (Figs 41 & 42). Since some asymptomatic patients may show similar features, a relationship between symptoms and manometric abnormalities is important.

Treatment Treatment with nitrates or calcium antagonists may produce symptomatic improvement in some patients. Pneumatic dilatation of the lower oesophageal sphincter may be useful in the minority. Only in patients with intractable symptoms should surgical intervention with a long myotomy be considered.

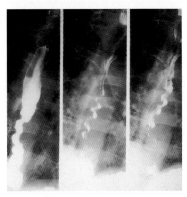

Fig. 40 Nutcracker oesophagus.

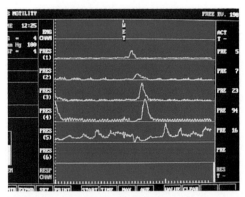

Fig. 41 Normal oesophageal manometry trace.

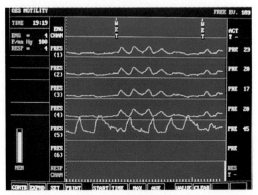

Fig. 42 Oesophageal manometry in oesophageal spasm.

Oesophageal varices

Structure: Oesophageal varices are most often found in patients with cirrhosis, but may occur with other causes of portal hypertension such as portal vein thrombosis. They may occur alone (Fig. 43) or in combination with gastric varices. Oesophageal varices are not simply large vessels, but rather distended normal oesophageal folds containing numerous dilated venules.

Bleeding: Although they are an important cause of upper gastrointestinal haemorrhage, it should be remembered that only a third of patients with oesophageal varices will ever bleed from these vessels. The risk of bleeding is greater in those with large vessels, particularly if cherry red spots are identified endoscopically.

Treatment The treatment of choice for bleeding oesophageal varices is endoscopic injection sclerotherapy or variceal ligation (Fig. 44) with the Sengstaken–Blakemore or Linton tube being used in those in whom bleeding cannot be controlled. Once bleeding has been controlled, sclerotherapy or variceal banding is usually repeated until variceal obliteration has been achieved. Sclerotherapy is not without its problems, which include ulceration, stricture formation and perforation. Transjugular intrahepatic portasystemic stent shunts (TIPSS) is a new technique which decompresses the portal system by creating a stented fistula between the portal and hepatic veins (Fig. 45) which is effective in controlling bleeding and preventing rebleeding. At present its main use is in the treatment of refractory bleeding from oesophageal varices, the treatment of bleeding from gastric varices and portal hypertensive gastropathy. Propranolol treatment should be considered in those with large varices which have not yet bled.

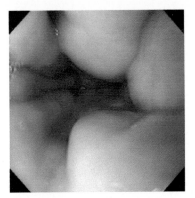

Fig. 43 Endoscopic appearance of oesophageal varices.

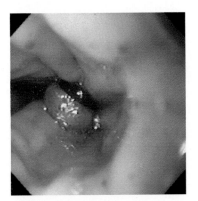

Fig. 44 Banded oesophageal varix.

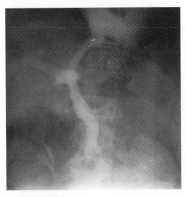

Fig. 45 TIPSS.

9 / Stomach

Peptic ulcer disease

The term peptic ulcer is primarily used for gastric and duodenal ulcers, but also includes oesophageal ulcers and stomal ulcers (Fig. 46). The overall incidence of peptic ulcer disease has been falling over the last 20 years, mainly in men. The frequency of gastric ulcers, particularly in the elderly, is increasing, whilst that of duodenal ulceration is falling.

Aetiology The aetiology of peptic ulcer disease has recently had to be rethought to incorporate gastric infection with *Helicobacter pylori* (Fig. 47). In duodenal ulceration the association with *H. pylori* is strong, such that in nearly all patients the organism can be found in the antrum and eradication of the organism almost invariable leads to ulcer healing. However, many patients have *H. pylori* infection and do not have peptic ulcer disease and such factors as high basal acid output and rapid gastric emptying are probably important. There is an association between blood group O and non-secretors of blood group antigens and duodenal ulcers. The association between *H. pylori* infection and gastric ulcers is not so strong and factors such as bile reflux and reduced protective mucosal factors are thought to be important.

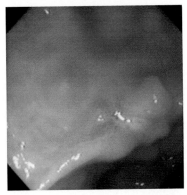

Fig. 46 Endoscopic appearance of a benign gastric ulcer.

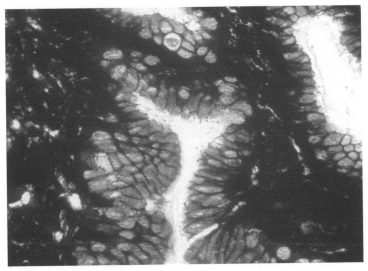

Fig. 47 Gastric biopsy showing *H. pylori*.

Peptic ulcer disease (cont.)

Clinical features
Clinical features of peptic ulcer disease include dyspepsia, often related to food intake. Epigastric pain that results in wakening during the night is highly typical of peptic ulceration. Ulcers may however be entirely silent or cause only minimal inconvenience and present with perforation or GI bleeding, manifest either as haematemesis or anaemia. Chronic ulceration may produce scarring and result in gastric outlet obstruction.

Investigation
The investigation of choice is fibre-optic endoscopy (Fig. 48) which allows not only identification of the ulcer, but also biopsy, which is essential to ensure that gastric ulcers are benign. It also allows antral biopsies to be taken to confirm the presence of *H. pylori* either histologically or by detection of urease in the tissue. Barium studies are less commonly used (Fig. 49).

Treatment
The treatment of choice for over 10 years for both gastric and duodenal ulcers has been H$_2$-antagonist therapy e.g. ranitidine or cimetidine. More recently the combination of these or omeprazole or the bismuth-containing agent De-Nol with an antibiotic combination such as amoxycillin and metronidazole has been shown to be both effective in eradicating *H. pylori* and healing the ulcers, and in reducing relapse, which, for duodenal ulcer disease in particular, is common after H$_2$-antagonist therapy alone.

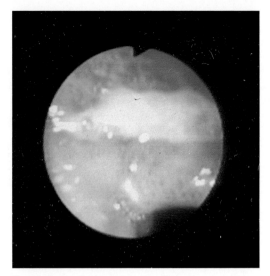

Fig. 48 Benign duodenal ulcer at endoscopy.

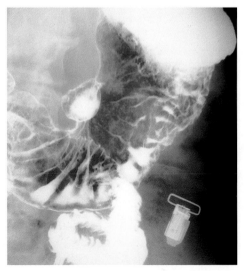

Fig. 49 Barium meal showing benign gastric ulcer.

Upper GI haemorrhage

Bleeding in the upper gastrointestinal tract results in haematemesis, the vomiting of recognisable blood and/or melaena—the passage of tarry-black faeces. If the bleeding rate is slow anaemia may be the sole presenting feature. True melaena nearly always follows bleeding proximal to the jejunum, although a black watery stool is not uncommon in patients with small intestinal or proximal colonic bleeding.

Aetiology   Approximately 50% of cases of upper GI haemorrhage are due to gastric or duodenal ulceration (Fig. 50), whilst bleeding from gastric erosions, Mallory-Weiss tear and oesophageal varices make up the majority of the remainder. Uncommon causes include gastric carcinoma, haemobilia, systemic diseases such as uraemia, connective tissue disorders and systemic infections and syndromes such as hereditary haemorrhagic telangiectasia and blue rubber-bleb naevi (Fig. 51).

History   Important aspects of the history include an estimate of the volume of blood loss, the time scale over which the bleeding has occurred, previous abdominal symptoms or history of peptic ulcer disease, recent ingestion of non-steroidal anti-inflammatory drugs including aspirin, retching or vomiting prior to the bleeding, alcohol abuse, known liver disease or weight loss suggestive of malignancy.

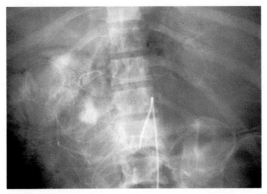

Fig. 50 Angiogram showing bleeding duodenal ulcer.

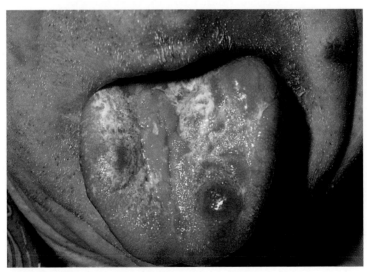

Fig. 51 Blue rubber-bleb naevi on the tongue.

Upper GI haemorrhage (cont.)

Examination

It is important to recognise haemodynamic disturbance indicating blood volume depletion e.g. systolic blood pressure less than 100 or heart rate over 100, stigmata of chronic liver disease, epigastric tenderness, abdominal distension with hyperactive bowel sounds suggesting large volume of blood in the intestine, splenomegaly or distended abdominal wall veins in portal hypertension, purpura as part of generalised bleeding disorder and nasopharyngeal bleeding which when swallowed may give rise to haematemesis and/or melaena.

Investigation and treatment

An urgent full blood count and urea and electrolyte profile should be obtained. It should be noted that the haemoglobin and haematocrit do not fall until haemodilution has occurred, which may take some hours. The blood urea is generally elevated with significant upper GI bleed and is disproportionate to the serum creatinine level. Upper gastrointestinal endoscopy should be undertaken early as it not only provides invaluable diagnostic information (Fig. 52), but in the case of bleeding peptic ulcers and varices allows injection sclerotherapy to be undertaken (Fig. 53). It is essential that before endoscopy is performed the patient should be adequately resuscitated and all patients admitted with suspected upper GI bleeding should have vascular access established early in their admission.

In patients who continue to bleed, in whom endoscopic treatment is not appropriate/possible or has failed, surgery should be undertaken early, particularly in the elderly.

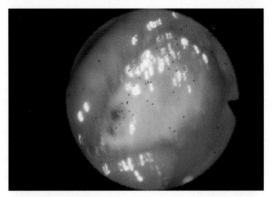

Fig. 52 Endoscopy showing duodenal ulcer with stigmata of recent haemorrhage.

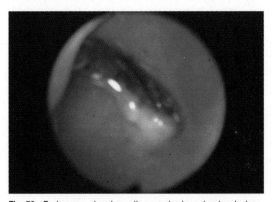

Fig. 53 Endoscopy showing adherent clot in a duodenal ulcer.

Gastric carcinoma

Frequency

Approximately 10 000 deaths per year occur in the UK from gastric carcinoma. The incidence is high in Japan and over recent years has been decreasing in Western countries.

Aetiology and risk factors

Risk factors include dried and salty foods, high fat diet, blood group A, pernicious anaemia, achlorhydria, smoking and male sex. It has long been thought that nitrates in the diet may be transformed into carcinogenic nitrosamines and such transformation is particularly likely in hypochlorhydric stomachs and in post-gastrectomy remnants. The role of *H. pylori* is uncertain.

Clinical features

These include abdominal pain, anorexia, weight loss, vomiting and dysphagia.

Diagnosis

The investigation of choice is gastroscopy, which allows not only visualisation of tumour, but biopsies to be taken (Fig. 54). Barium radiology is also a sensitive diagnostic tool, and features which suggest malignancy include rigidity of the gastric wall adjacent to an ulcer, an asymmetrical ulcer crater, greater curve ulcer and folds that do not radiate towards on ulcer crater (Fig. 55).

Treatment

Unfortunately the results of treatment of gastric cancer in Western countries are poor. It is primarily related to stage of the tumour at the time of diagnosis. In most cases nodal spread has already occurred at the time of diagnosis and the 5 year survival rate is less than 10% despite radical surgery. Early diagnosis as a result of screening programmes, which have been introduced in Japan, gives much better survival rates. In many cases treatment is directed mainly towards palliation i.e. the prevention of gastric outlet obstruction and dysphagia together with pain relief.

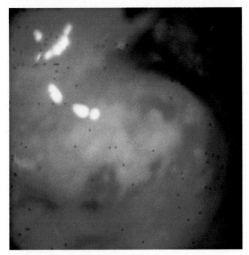

Fig. 54 Endoscopic appearance of gastric carcinoma.

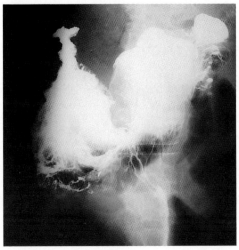

Fig. 55 Barium meal showing diffuse gastric carcinoma.

Ménétrièr's disease

This is an unusual condition characterised by hypertrophic gastric mucosa through which protein is lost. This may affect the entire body or fundus of the stomach or more localised areas, but not the antrum.

Clinical features
Patients are generally adults, often with oedema due to hypoproteinaemia. Other features may include nausea, vomiting and dyspepsia.

Investigations
The diagnosis may be suggested by barium radiology which shows giant mucosal folds (Fig. 56), or at endoscopy where folds remain obvious even after air distension and viscid mucus may be obvious (Fig. 57). Biopsies may or may not be diagnostic.

Treatment
Although steroid treatment and H_2-antagonist therapy have been suggested, surgery is generally required to prevent severe hypoproteinaemia.

Gastric varices

Aetiology
Gastric varices develop like oesophageal varices in patients with portal hypertension. They may develop in conjunction with oesophageal varices or in isolation, particularly in those with extrahepatic portal hypertension. Like oesophageal varices, they may be present for many years without bleeding, but once this has occurred their treatment is problematical. Compared with oesophageal varices they bleed less often but the bleeding is often more severe.

Treatment
Endoscopic sclerotherapy is reasonably effective in gastric varices which extend down the lesser curve connected to oesophageal varices. It is less successful in treating isolated varices in the cardia. In this situation surgical or transjugular intrahepatic portasystemic stent shunts are more likely to be required.

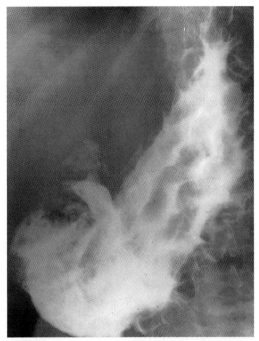
Fig. 56 Barium meal showing Ménétrièr's disease.

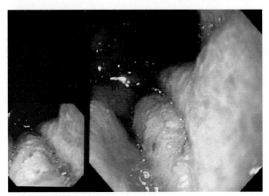
Fig. 57 Endoscopic appearance of Ménétrièr's disease.

Portal hypertensive gastropathy

This develops in many patients with portal hypertension and can be classified into mild forms where a characteristic snakeskin-like pattern is identifiable and severe forms where multiple red spots and contact bleeding are identifiable.

Clinical features The most common presentation is anaemia due to persistent oozing of blood from the gastric mucosa, which may or may not be demonstrable at endoscopy (Fig. 58).

Treatment The most effective treatment at present is probably with propranolol, which controls blood loss and reduces transfusion requirements in many patients. However, where this is unsuccessful, surgical or transjugular portal decompression may be required.

Ectopic varices

Occasionally varices may occur in extra-oesophagogastric sites—ectopic varices. They may arise in the duodenum (Fig. 59), colon, rectum, around an ileostomy (Fig. 60) or colostomy and vagina or bladder.

Clinical features They generally present with bleeding but less often with anorexia. Again, they are usually identified at endoscopy.

Treatment Sclerotherapy is less effective in their treatment than for oesophagogastric varices and surgical or transjugular portal decompression is often required.

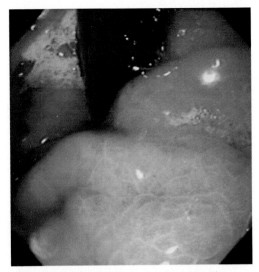

Fig. 58 Endoscopic appearance of portal gastropathy.

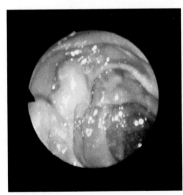

Fig. 59 Duodenal varices at endoscopy.

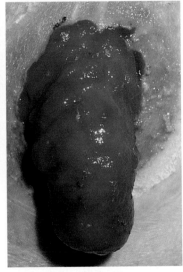

Fig. 60 Varices around an ileostomy.

10 / **Small intestine**

Coeliac disease

This immunologically mediated hypersensitivity to gluten occurs with a frequency of approximately 1 in 2000. The immunologically active component of gluten is thought to be gliadin. An important genetic association exists with an increased frequency of HLA B8 and DR3, but environmental factors are also important.

Clinical features
It is most commonly diagnosed in children who present with diarrhoea, steatorrhoea, weight loss or failure to thrive, although presentation in adults is not uncommon with diarrhoea or the consequences of malabsorption such as anaemia. Signs which may be found include mouth ulceration, peripheral oedema and occasionally dermatitis herpetiformis. This latter is characterised by an intensely itchy blistering skin eruption and responds to a gluten-free diet.

Investigations
Diagnosis should be made by jejunal or distal duodenal biopsy which demonstrates subtotal or total villus atrophy associated with a chronic inflammatory cell infiltrate (Figs 61 & 62). Investigations may also show anaemia and hypoalbuminaemia and the xylose tolerance test is generally abnormal.

Treatment
Gluten-containing foods, which include barley, wheat, oats and rye, should be withdrawn from the diet. A repeat biopsy after gluten withdrawal should show improvement in the small intestinal architecture.

Complications
An increase in incidence of small intestinal tumours especially lymphoma is well recognised, although the cause-effect relationship is less clear.

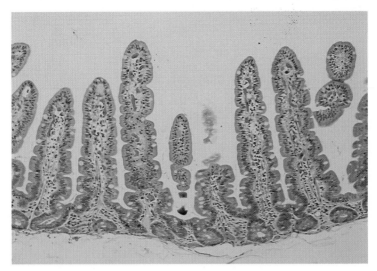

Fig. 61 Normal jejunal mucosa.

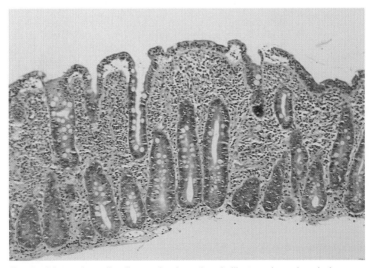

Fig. 62 Jejunum in coeliac disease showing subtotal villus atrophy and marked inflammatory infiltrate.

Small intestinal infection

Giardiasis

This infestation with *Giardia lamblia* is transmitted by the ingestion of infested water or the faecal-oral route.

Clinical features In many cases the infection may be asymptomatic. In those who develop symptoms they occur after a 1–3 week incubation period with diarrhoea, abdominal distension, pain, weight loss, nausea and vomiting. These usually only last a few days, but may continue for months. The diagnosis should be confirmed by microscopy of duodenal juice and faecal culture (Fig. 63), or identification of the organism in a distal duodenal or a jejunal biopsy (Fig. 64).

Treatment Treatment is with metronidazole, which will eradicate the organism in about 90% of patients. Alternative agents include tinidazole or quinacrine hydrochloride.

Coccidia

Coccidium parasites may infect the small intestine in humans and spread is by the faecal-oral route. In the proximal small intestine cysts release sporozoites which develop into trophozoites in the epithelium. The multiplication of the offspring from these damages the intestinal epithelium and results in partial and subtotal villus atrophy.

Clinical features Usually only a mild diarrhoreal illness develops a week or so after infection, but occasionally the infection may be severe with weight loss, colic, pyrexia and protracted diarrhoea. The diagnosis should be made by stool examination for coccidial ova or from jejunal biopsies.

Treatment Treatment is often not needed as it is usually self-limiting.

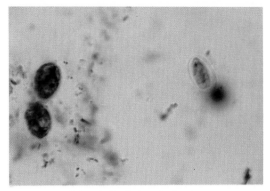

Fig. 63 Trophozoite of *Giardia intestinalis*.

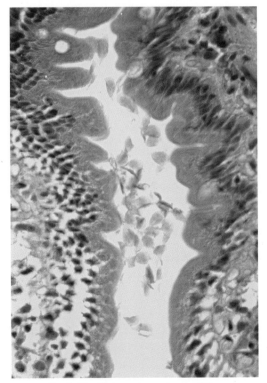

Fig. 64 *Giardia* identified on a lower duodenal biopsy

Small intestinal infection (cont.)

Typhoid and paratyphoid

These arise from infections with *Salmonella typhi* or *S. paratyphi* that are spread generally by food contamination. The bacilli multiply in the lymphoid tissue, generally in the ileum and this occasionally results in intestinal perforation or bleeding.

Clinical features The infection may be asymptomatic or characterised by mild abdominal pain. Diarrhoea or constipation may develop associated with a fever and a relative bradycardia. Diagnosis depends on isolating the organism from blood cultures at an early stage or from stool.

Treatment Treatment is with chloramphenicol, ampicillin or co-trimoxazole.

Cryptosporidium

Clinical features This protozoan produces diarrhoea, malabsorption, weight loss, fever and abdominal pain. Diagnosis should be by stool culture looking for oocytes and small bowel biopsy (Fig. 65).

Infection is commoner in those who are immunosuppressed.

Treatment Treatment should be with spiramycin along with anti-diarrhoeal agents.

Helminth infestations

The commonest helminth infestations of the small intestine are with ascarids (Fig. 66) and hookworms (*Ancylostoma duodenale* and *Necator americanus*).

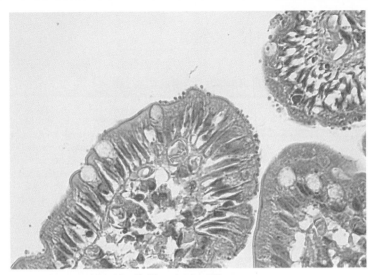

Fig. 65 *Cryptosporidium* identified in a duodenal biopsy.

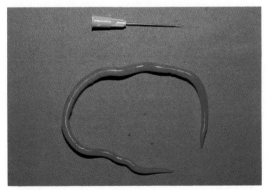

Fig. 66 *Ascaris lumbricoides.*

Small intestinal infection (cont.)

Tuberculosis

This is rare in Western but common in developing countries. Presentation is with weight loss, fever, abdominal pain and diarrhoea. The commonest site involved is the ileocaecal region and it must be differentiated from Crohn's disease and malignancy (Fig. 67).

Bacterial overgrowth

This may occur as a result of structural abnormality, motility disorders or immunological deficiency. Common causes include gastric surgery, pernicious anaemia, enteroanastomosis, duodenal or jejunal diverticulae (Fig. 68), diabetic neuropathy and scleroderma.

Clinical features
The commonest presentation is with anaemia due to vitamin B12 deficiency and less often folate deficiency. Other features include steatorrhoea, diarrhoea and oedema due to hypoproteinaemia. Diagnosis may be made by reversal of malabsorption by treatment with broad-spectrum antibiotics or by positive glycocholic acid breath test.

Treatment
Treatment should be with antibiotics, vitamin supplements or surgery where appropriate.

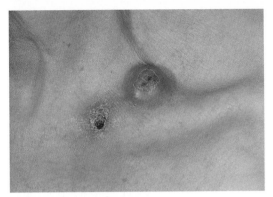

Fig. 67 Tuberculous neck sinus.

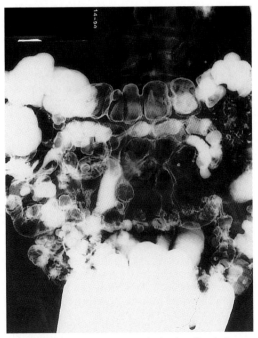

Fig. 68 Small bowel follow-through showing diverticulae.

Whipple's disease (intestinal lipodystrophy)
This is a rare disorder of unknown aetiology which is more common in males than females.

Clinical features
Clinical features include malabsorption, weight loss, lymphadenopathy, abdominal pain, a migratory polyarthritis often involving the knees or ankles, pyrexia, peripheral oedema, abdominal distension or tenderness and skin pigmentation. The diagnosis is made by small intestinal biopsy that shows partial or subtotal villus atrophy with foamy-looking macrophages filled with PAS-positive granules (Fig. 69). Rod-shaped bacteria may be seen just below the epithelium.

Treatment
Prolonged treatment with tetracycline for at least 12 months is recommended.

Lymphoma of the small intestine

Lymphoma is the commonest tumour of the small intestine. Primary lymphomas arise within the mucosa and submucosa of the intestine and involve regional lymph nodes secondarily. This tumour arises most often in the distal ileum and least frequently in the proximal jejunum.

Clinical features
The condition is commoner in males and arises usually in the middle-aged and elderly. Presenting features include abdominal pain, nausea, vomiting, intestinal bleeding, weight loss and anaemia. Finger clubbing is uncommon except in the 'Mediterranean type' lymphoma. Malabsorption is a common presenting feature in this latter variant.

Diagnosis
The diagnosis is usually made on a barium follow-through examination and may be difficult to differentiate from Crohn's disease or other malignancies. Like Crohn's disease, multiple areas of involvement may be demonstrated as may fistulae (Figs 70 & 71).

Treatment
Treatment is usually surgical with or without postoperative radiotherapy.

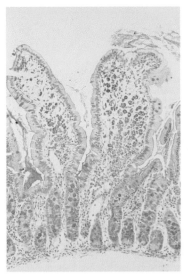

Fig. 69 Whipple's disease. PAS-positive macrophages are clearly seen.

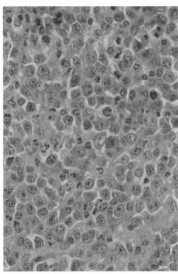

Fig. 70 Microscopic appearance of small bowel lymphoma.

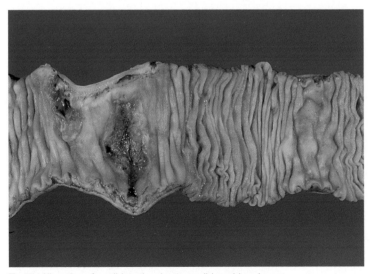

Fig. 71 Ulceration of small intestine due to small bowel lymphoma.

Meckel's diverticulum

This congenital abnormality occurs in approximately 2% of the population. It is the remnant of the vitelline duct and occurs on the anti-mesenteric border of the ileum, approximately 2 feet from the ileocaecal valve. Gastric mucosa occurs in approximately 50% and pancreatic tissue in approximately 5%.

Clinical features In many cases Meckel's diverticulum is asymptomatic and bleeding is the most common complication due to ulceration secondary to acid secretion from the ectopic gastric mucosa. The diagnosis should be considered in patients where the source of gastrointestinal haemorrhage cannot be found.

Investigations The diagnosis is usually made by radionuclide scanning or angiography. Another complication that may arise is intussusception or volvulus around the fibrous cord that connects the diverticulum to the umbilicus in approximately 25% of cases. Inflammation of the diverticulum may give rise to a clinical picture that simulates acute appendicitis or may perforate.

Treatment Surgery is indicated (Fig. 72) only in cases where complications have arisen.

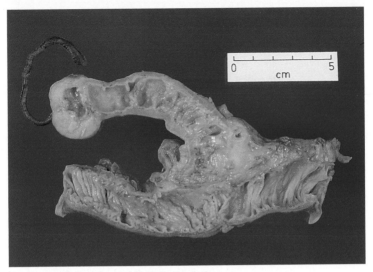

Fig. 72 Resected specimen of Meckel's diverticulum.

11 / Biliary tract

Primary biliary cirrhosis

Definitions This disease of unknown aetiology results in granulomatous destructive cholangitis.

Clinical features Approximately 90% of patients are female and usually present with itch which may or may not be associated with jaundice. Another common presentation is the finding of cholestatic liver function tests i.e. glutamyl transferase and alkaline phosphatase during routine biochemical screening. Skin xanthomas occur, especially over the eyelids (xanthelasma palpabarum). Primary biliary cirrhosis may be associated with osteomalacia, osteoporosis and spontaneous fractures and other autoimmune diseases, the sicca syndrome with xerostomia and keratoconjunctivitis sicca are particularly common. The latter is detected by Schirmer's test. Other signs are those of portal hypertension e.g. caput medusa (Fig. 73) or decompensated cirrhosis.

Diagnosis The following features are usually present: antimitochondrial antibodies, cholestatic liver function tests, normal biliary system on ultrasound or ERCP and cholestatic histology with peribiliary inflammation and granulomata, with or without fibrosis (Fig. 74).

Treatment Primary biliary cirrhosis runs a variable course which may ultimately result in hepatic cirrhosis, with its associated complications—transplantation may then be indicated. Ursodeoxycholic acid results in biochemical improvement.

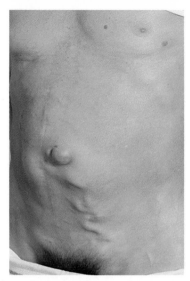

Fig. 73 Caput medusa.

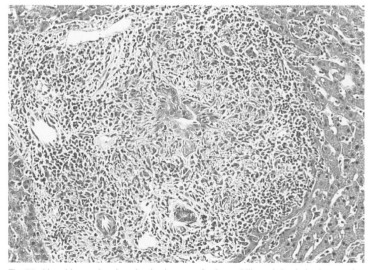

Fig. 74 Liver biopsy showing classic changes of primary biliary cirrhosis in the portal tracts.

Primary sclerosing cholangitis

This condition can affect both the intrahepatic and extrahepatic biliary tree.

Aetiology It is of unknown aetiology and is associated with inflammatory bowel disease. Sclerosing cholangitis can also occur in patients with AIDS, graft versus host disease, parasitic and bacterial infection and hepatic arterial chemotherapy.

Clinical features Patients may present with cholangitis, fever and right upper quadrant pain. Some present with established cirrhosis and its associated complications. Sclerosing cholangitis is increasingly identified in patients with inflammatory bowel disease, whilst they are asymptomatic, by finding elevation of alkaline phosphatase and gamma glutamyl transferase.

Investigations A liver biopsy shows characteristic concentric collagen deposition around intrahepatic bile ducts. Endoscopic retrograde cholangiography reveals irregular stricturing which can affect both the intrahepatic and extrahepatic biliary tree (Figs 75 & 76).

Treatment There is no specific treatment, but liver transplantation may be indicated. The incidence of cholangiocarcinoma is increased in primary sclerosing cholangitis.

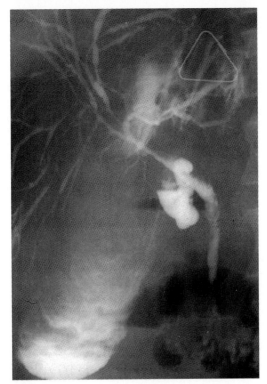

Fig. 75 Primary sclerosing cholangitis.

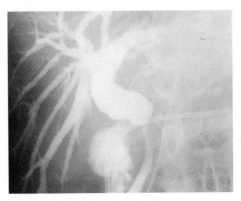

Fig. 76 Primary sclerosing cholangitis.

Cystic disease of the liver

The cysts may be single or multiple. Single cysts are usually benign, but may arise from infection with hydatid (Fig. 77). Polycystic renal disease can be associated with multiple liver cysts. These arise from defective development of the intrahepatic bile ducts. The clinical symptoms are predominantly related to the renal disease, although some patients may complain of chronic abdominal pain with acute exacerbation secondary to haemorrhage or infection of the cysts.

Choledochal cysts

Dilatation of the common bile duct occurs which may present in infants as prolonged cholestasis or in adults with intermittent jaundice, pain and a palpable abdominal mass. Treatment is by surgical excision.

Biliary strictures

Aetiology These may be either benign or malignant (Fig. 78). Benign strictures are usually iatrogenic following surgical trauma or due to ischaemia or sclerosing cholangitis. Bile duct tumours are more common in patients with sclerosing cholangitis, polycystic liver disease, choledochal cysts and chronic infection with the liver fluke *Clonorchis sinensis*.

Clinical features Patients present with jaundice, itch and abdominal pain. Symptoms include recurrent cholangitis with fever, jaundice and abdominal pain which is treated with antibiotics.

Treatment A benign stricture may be dilated at ERCP and a stent inserted. Reconstructive surgery may however be required. Malignant biliary strictures are managed with palliative treatment following insertion of biliary stents either percutaneously or at ERCP (Fig. 79). Surgical resection is rarely possible.

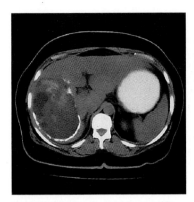

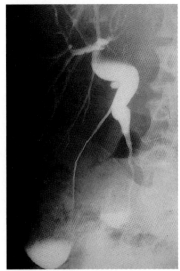

Fig. 77 Hydatid cyst of the liver on CT scan.

Fig. 78 Percutaneous transhepatic cholangiogram showing a benign stricture of the common bile duct.

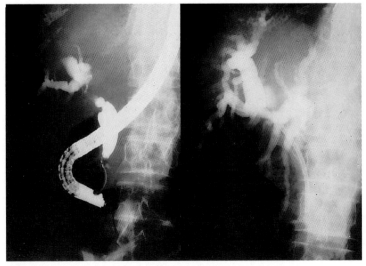

Fig. 79 ERCP stenting of malignant biliary stricture.

12 / **Gallbladder**

Gallstones

Aetiology

These may be of three main types: cholesterol stones, black stones of bilirubin and brown stones of calcium salts. Black bilirubin-containing stones are associated with chronic haemolysis, brown stones are often associated with chronic biliary infection. Cholesterol stones are more common in the elderly, women, obese patients and following ileal resection and prolonged cholestyramine therapy.

Clinical features

Gallstones may obstruct the cystic duct, resulting in acute cholecystitis with abdominal pain and fever and may produce chronic cholecystitis with chronic abdominal pain. Acute cholecystitis may be complicated by gangrene and perforation of the gallbladder or empyema. Gallstones may migrate and obstruct the common bile duct, resulting in ascending cholangitis with jaundice, fever and abdominal pain.

Diagnosis

Gallstones may be identified by ultrasound (Fig. 80). In obstructive jaundice dilated intrahepatic bile ducts may be identified (Fig. 81). ERCP is also useful and may allow definitive treatment (Fig. 82).

Treatment

Treatment is by cholecystectomy, now usually undertaken laparoscopically. Medical dissolution therapy is only rarely considered but may be used as an adjunct when lithotripsy has been used to disintegrate gallstones. Patients with stones in the common bile duct are treated with antibiotics, ERCP with endoscopic sphincterotomy, or surgical exploration and cholecystectomy.

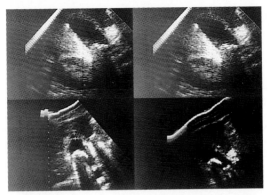

Fig. 80 Ultrasound showing gallstones with acoustic shadow behind the stones.

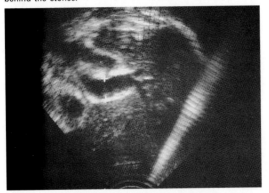

Fig. 81 Ultrasound showing dilated bile ducts in obstructive jaundice secondary to common duct stones.

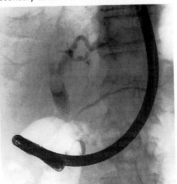

Fig. 82 ERCP showing common duct stones.

13 / Pancreas

Acute pancreatitis

Aetiology   Acute inflammation of the pancreas is most commonly caused by alcohol excess or gallstones. It can also be associated with viral infection, ingestion of certain drugs e.g. thiazide diuretics, or more rarely with hypercalcaemia or hyperlipidaemia.

Clinical features   Patients present with abdominal pain and, if pancreatitis is severe, with shock, oliguria and multiple organ failure. Severe cases are associated with hypocalcaemia, clinically detectable by Chvostek's or Trousseau's sign and retroperitoneal haemorrhage producing bruising around the umbilicus (Cullen's sign) or in the flanks (Gray-Turner's sign) (Fig. 84). High serum amylase or immunoreactive trypsin occur in acute cases.

Treatment   Treatment is supportive, early ERCP with endoscopic sphincterotomy is beneficial in those caused by gallstones. Surgical necrosectomy may be undertaken in patients with pancreatic necrosis. Development of a pseudocyst (Fig. 83) is treated with surgical or endoscopic drainage.

Chronic pancreatitis

Aetiology   Chronic pancreatitis (Fig. 85) is most commonly caused by alcohol ingestion. Other causes include tropical pancreatitis, hypoparathyroidism, hereditary and idiopathic forms.

Clinical features   Patients present with chronic abdominal pain which often radiates to the back and is relieved by sitting forward. In severe cases there is malabsorption secondary to exocrine pancreatic insufficiency and diabetes mellitus due to endocrine insufficiency.

Treatment   Treatment includes lifelong abstinence from alcohol, analgesics, nerve blocks and surgical intervention to relieve the abdominal pain. Malabsorption is treated by pancreatic enzyme supplements and diabetes requires insulin therapy.

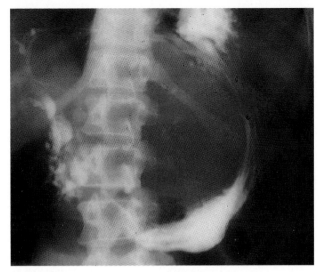

Fig. 83 Barium meal showing pancreatic pseudocyst.

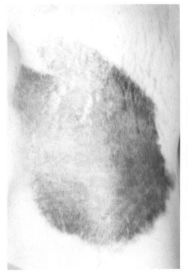

Fig. 84 Gray-Turner's sign.

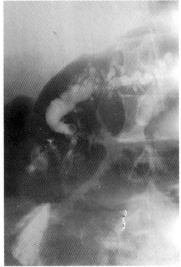

Fig. 85 Chronic calcific pancreatitis.

Pancreatic carcinoma

Aetiology Adenocarcinoma most often arises within the head of the pancreas gland. It is associated with male sex, smoking and heavy alcohol consumption.

Clinical features Patients can present with abdominal pain, profound weight loss and jaundice if the common bile duct is involved. Chronic blood loss from an ampullary tumour may produce a characteristic silvery stool. Diagnosis is by ultrasound with guided biopsy, CT scanning (Fig. 86) and angiography.

Treatment Surgical resection is the only possible curative treatment and is especially useful in ampullary tumours. Palliative treatment includes surgical bypass of the duodenum and biliary tree or stenting through the tumour, either percutaneously or endoscopically (Fig. 87). The prognosis is poor with most patients dying within 1 year of diagnosis.

Pancreatic endocrine tumours

These uncommon tumours can secrete gastrin with the development of Zollinger-Ellison syndrome, characterised by resistant peptic ulceration. Vasoactive intestinal peptide-secreting tumours produce the Werner-Morrison syndrome with hypokalaemia, achlorhydria and watery diarrhoea. Glucagon-secreting tumours produce a characteristic skin rash and diabetes and insulin-secreting tumours produce recurrent episodes of hypoglycaemia.

Treatment Treatment for these tumours is by surgical resection, although in Zollinger-Ellison syndrome high dose H_2 antagonists or omeprazole therapy may be useful. Octreotide therapy is also effective in a variety of pancreatic tumours.

Cystic fibrosis

Cystic fibrosis is inherited as an autosomal recessive trait. It can affect the pancreas with associated malabsorption and steatorrhoea. Symptoms can be controlled with oral pancreatic enzyme supplements.

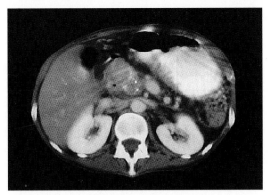

Fig. 86 CT scan showing a mass in the head of the pancreas.

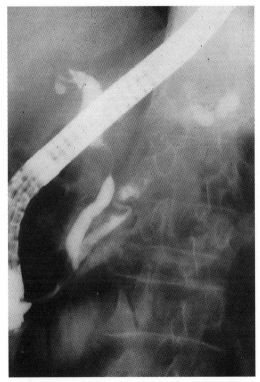

Fig. 87 ERCP showing obstruction secondary to pancreatic cancer. Stenting will relieve the biliary obstruction.

14 / Liver

Fulminant liver failure

Definition   This is defined as the development of hepatic encephalopathy within 8 weeks of the onset of symptoms in a patient with previously normal liver function.

Aetiology   It has many causes, the most common in the UK is paracetamol overdosage. Hepatitis A (rarely), hepatitis B and other viruses can produce fulminant liver failure, which is more common in Europe. Other causes include toxins (e.g. *Amanita phalloides*), acute fatty liver of pregnancy and Budd-Chiari syndrome.

Clinical features   Characteristically after ingestion of more than 10–15 g of paracetamol the patient develops jaundice, coagulopathy, hypoglycaemia, hepatic encephalopathy and cerebral oedema (Fig. 88) within 3 days of the overdose. As paracetamol is also nephrotoxic, acute renal failure commonly accompanies the hepatic necrosis.

Treatment   Skilled intensive medical and nursing care is required (Fig. 89). Liver transplantation is indicated in certain patients with a predicted poor prognosis.

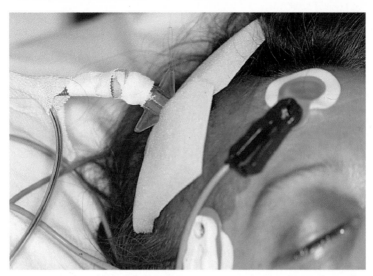

Fig. 88 Intracranial pressure monitor to allow early diagnosis of cerebral oedema and intracranial hypertension.

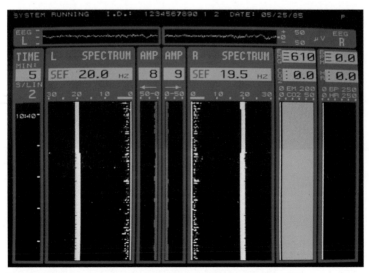

Fig. 89 Cerebrotrack monitor tracing in a patient with fulminant liver failure.

Chronic active hepatitis

Definition In liver biopsies piecemeal necrosis of hepatocytes occurs around the limiting plate of the portal tracts (Fig. 90), this results in cirrhosis if prolonged.

Aetiology May be produced by infection with hepatitis B (Figs 91 & 92) or C or occur in patients with Wilson's disease, alpha-l-antitrypsin deficiency (Fig. 93) and chronic alcoholism. Reactions to alpha-methyl-dopa and isoniazid may induce chronic active hepatitis. One of the largest groups of causes is so-called autoimmune or 'lupoid' hepatitis.

Clinical features This is dependent on the aetiology of the chronic active hepatitis. Patients may present with asymptomatic abnormal serum biochemical tests (elevated AST, ALT), fatigue, jaundice or decompensated cirrhosis or uncommonly fulminant liver failure.

Diagnosis Liver biopsy is essential in diagnosis. The underlying aetiology may be suggested by finding positive autoantibodies in autoimmune chronic active hepatitis (positive antinuclear factor and anti-smooth muscle antibody), reduced serum ceruloplasmin and increased urinary copper in Wilson's disease, reduced serum alpha-l-antitrypsin level and abnormal phenotype in patients with alpha-l-antitrypsin deficiency and in viral hepatitis the presence of hepatitis B surface antigen and hepatitis Be antigen or antibody to hepatitis C in the blood.

Treatment Viral hepatitis may be treated by interferon therapy with improvement in 25–50% of cases. Autoimmune chronic active hepatitis is treated with steroids and other immunosuppressive therapy. Wilson's disease is treated by chelating agents, most commonly D-penicillamine.

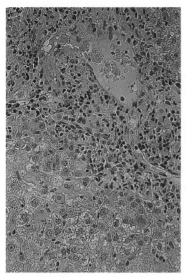

Fig. 90 Chronic active hepatitis.

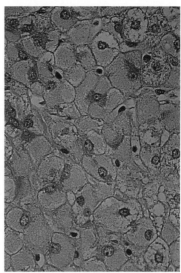

Fig. 91 Ground glass appearance of hepatocytes in a patient with hepatitis B.

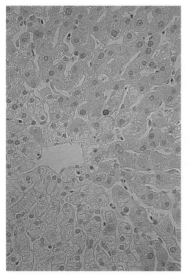

Fig. 92 Immunohistochemical staining for hepatitis B surface antigen expressed in hepatocytes.

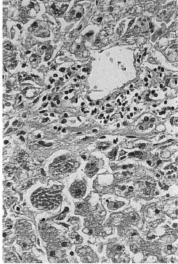

Fig. 93 PAS-positive cells in a patient with alpha-1-antitrypsin deficiency.

Cirrhosis

Definitions   Cirrhosis is a disease characterised by destruction of liver cells with fibrosis, subsequent nodular transformation and proliferation of the remaining hepatocytes. This may be differentiated laparoscopically (Fig. 94) or histologically (Fig. 95) into macro-and micro-nodular forms.

Aetiology   Hepatic cirrhosis, like chronic active hepatitis, has multiple causes including those listed under chronic active hepatitis, namely, chronic viral infection with B or C viruses, autoimmune chronic active hepatitis, Wilson's disease, alpha-l-antitrypsin deficiency and excess alcohol consumption. Other causes of cirrhosis include reactions to drugs (e.g. methotrexate), infection with schistosomiasis, primary biliary cirrhosis, haemochromatosis, sclerosing cholangitis, chronic heart failure, Budd-Chiari syndrome and certain inborn errors of metabolism.

Clinical features   Patients may present with the symptoms of decompensated cirrhosis; hepatic encephalopathy, ascites, variceal haemorrhage or hepatocellular carcinoma. Alternatively, patients may have abnormal liver function tests at biochemical screening, but are completely asymptomatic.

Endocrine abnormalities: Gynaecomastia, testicular atrophy and female distribution of body hair is common in male patients with cirrhosis, particularly alcoholic cirrhosis. In patients with alcoholic cirrhosis there may be facial features suggestive of Cushing's disease (pseudo-Cushing's syndrome) which must be differentiated from bilateral parotid swelling which occurs in alcoholic cirrhosis. In women erratic menstruation and breast atrophy occurs.

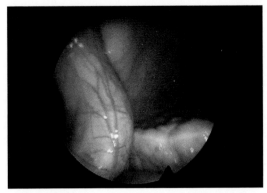

Fig. 94 Laparoscopy showing macronodular cirrhosis of the liver and a large varix on the falciform ligament.

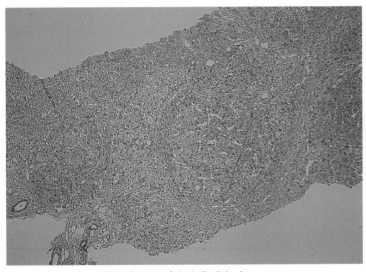

Fig. 95 Liver biopsy showing features of alcoholic cirrhosis.

Cirrhosis (cont.)

Portal hypertension

Aetiology   Although the most common cause of portal hypertension is hepatic cirrhosis, it can occur because of portal vein obstruction either extrahepatic—secondary to thrombosis or malignancy, or intrahepatic—due to congenital fibrosis or schistosomiasis.

Clinical features   The patients develop rectal or anal varices or, more commonly, varices within the oesophagus which may haemorrhage, the most dramatic presentation of patients with portal hypertension. A caput medusa around the umbilicus may be observed. Splenomegaly is palpable.

Diagnosis   Portal hypertension can be diagnosed by measuring the wedged hepatic venous or portal vein pressure. More commonly the presence of portal hypertension can be inferred by the observation of varices at an endoscopic examination of the oesophagus (Fig. 96).

Treatment   Portal pressure may be reduced acutely with vasoactive drugs such as vasopressin, glypressin or somatostatin. Prolonged oral treatment with propranolol and nitrates can chronically reduce portal pressure. The treatment of variceal bleeding involves endoscopy, with injection sclerotherapy with sclerosants or tissue adhesives. If this fails, balloon tamponade using a Sengstaken-Blakemore or Minnesota tube may provide temporary benefit (Fig. 97). More recently the introduction of transjugular intrahepatic portasystemic stent shunts has found application in the treatment of portal hypertension. Surgically fashioned portal systemic shunts have fallen out of favour because of the high operative mortality in poor risk cases and the occurrence of encephalopathy.

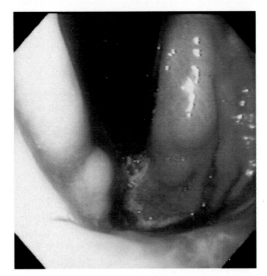

Fig. 96 Endoscopic appearance of gastric varices.

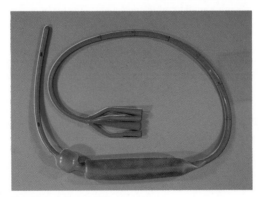

Fig. 97 Four-lumen Minnesota tube.

Ascites

Aetiology Ascites is the development of fluid within the abdominal cavity. This may be a transudate (protein concentration less than 30 g/l) or an exudate (protein concentration greater than 30 g/l). A transudate is most commonly associated with hepatic cirrhosis although it may also be caused by constrictive pericarditis, Budd-Chiari syndrome or pancreatitis. Exudative ascites is most commonly associated with infection, e.g. tuberculosis or malignancy.

Clinical features Ascites may develop insidiously or suddenly with variable swelling of the abdomen (Fig. 98). This may be associated with peripheral oedema or pleural effusions, most commonly right-sided.

Diagnosis Diagnostic paracentesis reveals the presence of fluid within the abdomen (Fig. 99), allows the differentiation between an exudate and transudate, bacteriological and cytological examination of the fluid and the measurement of amylase (high in pancreatic ascites). Ultrasound is able to detect the presence of fluid within the abdomen that is not obvious clinically and may also suggest possible aetiology, for example, identification of an ovarian tumour.

Treatment Treatment of ascites associated with cirrhosis is by salt restriction, fluid restriction and diuretic therapy (spironolactone). Occasionally these therapies do not work and the patient may require a therapeutic paracentesis or the insertion of a peritoneal-venous shunt.

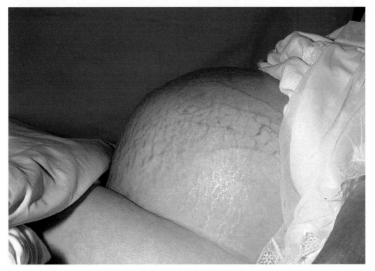

Fig. 98 Abdominal swelling in ascites.

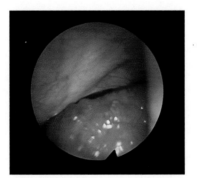

Fig. 99 Laparoscopy showing hepatic cirrhosis and ascites.

Hepatic encephalopathy

Definition   Hepatic encephalopathy is difficult to define into a single entity as it affects almost all cerebral functions. There is disturbed consciousness with inversion of the sleep rhythm and nightmares; personality changes and intellectual deterioration occur and slowing or slurring of the speech.

Aetiology   Hepatic encephalopathy may be caused by acute liver failure as discussed above. It also occurs in patients with cirrhosis and can be precipitated by excessive diuretic therapy, haemorrhage, paracentesis, diarrhoea, vomiting, sedative treatment, infections, drugs and toxins (including alcohol) and surgical treatment. Rarely a chronic portal systemic encephalopathy syndrome occurs with no obvious precipitant.

Diagnosis   The observation of changes in the patients' personality or mental functions may be associated with deterioration in their writing and failure to reproduce simple drawings (constructional apraxia) (Fig. 100). A flapping tremor (asterixis) may be elicited when the patients stretch their arms out, extending their wrists back. A similar flapping tremor may be elicited in the feet. There is hyperreflexia with extensor plantar responses in severe cases. Chronic encephalopathy may be characterised by abnormal facial movements and gait ataxia. An ECG would show typically increased slow wave activity (Fig. 101).

Treatment   Treatment is by reversing any precipitant, a reduced protein diet and treatment with lactulose.

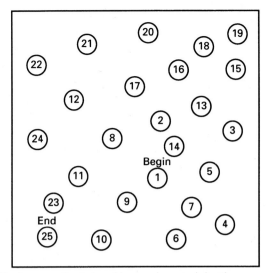

Fig. 100 Number connection test used in assessing encephalopathy.

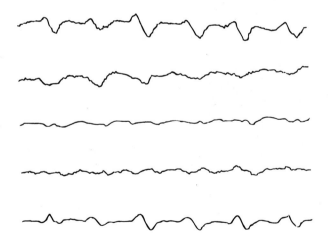

Fig. 101 Electroencephalograph showing excess slow wave activity in a patient with encephalopathy.

Liver tumours

Liver tumours may be benign, including haemangiomas, adenomas and focal nodular hyperplasia. Malignant liver tumours are most commonly metastatic from extrahepatic sites, although primary liver cancer (hepatocellular carcinoma) can complicate cirrhosis. Angiosarcomas and lymphomas of the liver are rare. Tumours arising from the bile ducts have been discussed previously.

Benign liver tumours

Angiomas

These tumours may be identified incidentally on ultrasound or a CT examination (Figs 102 & 103). Occasionally because of bleeding there is pain. Pressure on adjacent structures with large angiomas may also result in symptoms. No treatment is usually necessary although resection may be undertaken for large tumours (Fig. 104) or if there is rapid expansion.

Hepatic adenomas

These may also be identified incidentally on ultrasound examination. They may present as right upper quadrant masses or with acute intraperitoneal haemorrhage. They are treated by resection.

Focal nodular hyperplasia

This may present as a mass lesion with pressure on surrounding structures or be identified incidentally on ultrasound or CT examination. Characteristically there is a central stellate scar (Fig. 105). A problem with focal nodular hyperplasia is that it may be mistakenly diagnosed as cirrhosis.

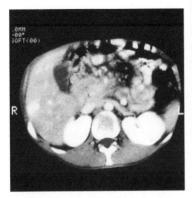

Fig. 102 CT scan post-contrast showing peripheral angioma.

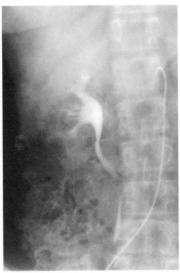

Fig. 103 Angiogram showing hepatic angioma.

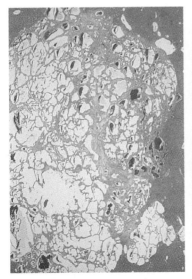

Fig. 104 Small angioma removed incidentally during hepatic resection.

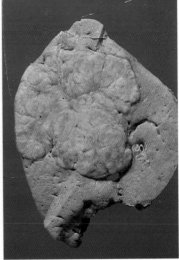

Fig. 105 Focal nodular hyperplasia.

Liver tumours (cont.)

Hepatocellular carcinoma

Aetiology It is uncommon to find hepatocellular carcinoma in patients who do not have cirrhosis. Hepatoma is particularly associated with post-viral cirrhosis and may complicate aflatoxin ingestion.

Clinical features Usually a deterioration occurs in patients with known cirrhosis resulting in ascites, abdominal pain, anorexia and weight loss. Symptoms may also be due to secondary spread, most typically to the lungs, bone or brain.

Diagnosis A high serum alphafetoprotein (AFP) is very suggestive of hepatocellular carcinoma. Further localisation of the tumour is by ultrasound, CT scan and angiography (Fig. 106). These imaging techniques can be used to direct a biopsy (Figs 107 & 108).

Treatment Identification of tumours that are small offers the best hope of cure by surgical resection. Liver transplantation may be indicated when there is no evidence of extrahepatic spread. Larger tumours can be treated by injection of ethanol into the tumour (ethanol tumour necrosis) or embolisation with local chemotherapy. Screening patients with cirrhosis by measurement of the AFP may result in the early detection of hepatocellular carcinoma. Prophylactic immunisation with hepatitis B vaccine in high prevalence areas may reduce the incidence of this tumour and this is also one of the long-term goals of treatment of chronic hepatitis B and C with interferon.

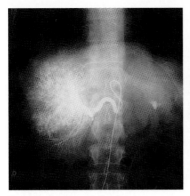

Fig. 106 Angiogram showing hepatocellular carcinoma.

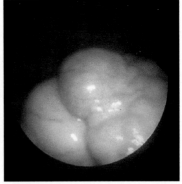

Fig. 107 Laparoscopy showing a prominent nodule, which on biopsy proved to be hepatocellular carcinoma.

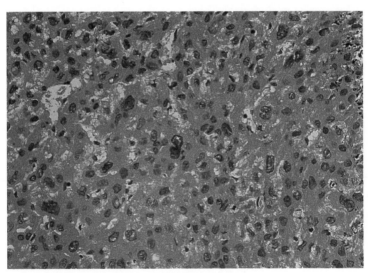

Fig. 108 Histological appearance of hepatocellular carcinoma.

Liver tumours (cont.)

Hepatic metastases

Aetiology   Liver is a common site for blood-borne metastases most commonly from stomach, breast, lung and those arising within organs drained by the portal vein.

Clinical features   These may be due to the hepatic metastases which can produce pain, or the primary tumour, or both. Often the patients are anorexic with weight loss and malaise. The liver is enlarged and irregular, occasionally umbilicated nodules can be felt. Ascites suggests peritoneal involvement.

Diagnosis   Ultrasound or CT scanning (Fig. 109) may show widespread metastases in the liver, and elevated serum carcinoembryonic antigen is suggestive of an intestinal origin for the tumour. Liver biopsy undertaken percutaneously, laparoscopically (Fig. 110) or under guidance with ultrasound or CT is frequently diagnostic.

Therapy   Single or multiple tumours affecting one lobe of the liver may be treated by resection. More commonly multiple metastases are present. Treatments with chemotherapy have produced variable results.

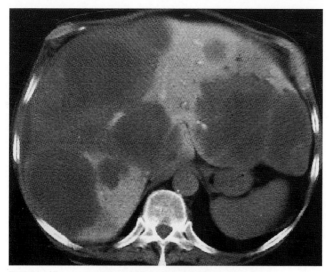

Fig. 109 CT scan showing multiple liver metastases.

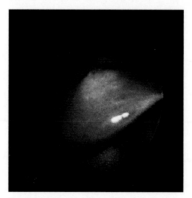

Fig. 110 Laparoscopic appearance of a hepatic metastasis from colonic carcinoma.

15 / **Lower GI tract**

Appendix inflammation

Clinical features   Acute inflammation of the appendix presents with central abdominal pain which shifts after several hours to localised pain with peritonism in the right iliac fossa. There may be associated fever, vomiting and diarrhoea dependent on the site of the appendix. Acute appendicitis may mimic Crohn's disease of the ileocaecal region, mesenteric adenitis or torsion of a Meckel's diverticulum.

Treatment   Treatment is with appendicectomy (Figs 111 & 112).

Carcinoma and carcinoid

Aetiology   Carcinoid of the appendix is the most common tumour of the appendix (Figs 113 & 114). It is benign with metastases and carcinoid syndrome only rarely being observed. Carcinoma of the appendix is a much less common condition.

Clinical features   Patients present with symptoms similar to acute appendicitis. It is unusual for carcinoid of the appendix to metastasise and so carcinoid syndrome is rare.

Treatment   Treatment is with appendicectomy.

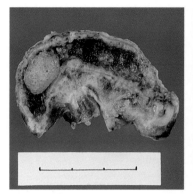

Fig. 111 Macroscopic appearances of acute appendicitis with an impacted faecalith.

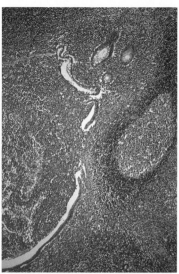

Fig. 112 Histological features of acute appendicitis.

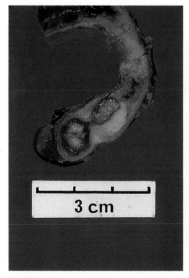

3 cm

Fig. 113 Macroscopic appearance of carcinoid of the appendix.

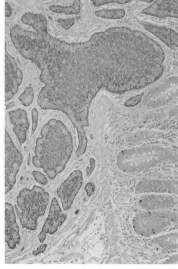

Fig. 114 Histological features of carcinoid tumour.

Diseases of the colon

Infection
The colon may be infected directly by a variety of microorganisms.

Clinical features

Shigellae and amoebae (Fig. 115) produce a dysentery-like syndrome with fever, abdominal pain and bloody diarrhoea. This needs to be differentiated from inflammatory bowel disease by stool culture, rectal biopsy or serological testing.

Treatment

Treatment is with appropriate antibiotic therapy.

Pseudomembranous colitis
This acute diarrhoeal illness occurs following antibiotic therapy and is due to infection with a toxin-producing strain of *Clostridium difficile*. Histological examination of a rectal biopsy or resected specimen shows typical changes (Fig. 116).

Treatment

Treatment is with oral vancomycin or metronidazole. Toxic dilatation rarely occurs and requires colectomy.

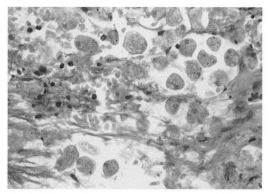

Fig. 115 Histological features of *Entamoeba histolytica* infection. The amoebae are clearly seen.

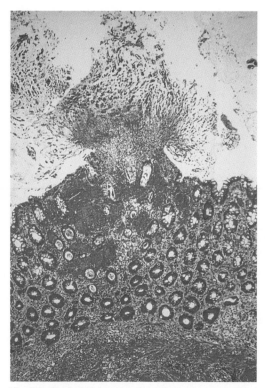

Fig. 116 Histological features of pseudomembranous colitis.

Inflammatory bowel disease

Definition Inflammatory bowel disease is a chronic non-specific
inflammatory condition of the bowel (Fig. 117) which
on clinical and pathological grounds may be
differentiated into two main forms.
Crohn's disease can involve any part of the
gastrointestinal tract from the mouth to the anus (Fig.
118). *Ulcerative colitis* is limited to the large bowel,
although there may be 'backwash ileitis' affecting the
terminal ileum. There are other uncommon colitides
described which may present in similar ways to
inflammatory bowel disease and are usually diagnosed
only on biopsy. In *microscopic colitis* there are no
macroscopic features of inflammation which are
readily seen on rectal biopsy. In *collagenous colitis*
there is a characteristic band of collagen just beneath
the mucosa (Fig. 119).

Epidemiology Crohn's disease affects 7–8 people per 100 000
whereas ulcerative colitis affects 10–12 per 100 000.
Inflammatory bowel disease is more common in first
degree relatives of affected patients and has a peak
incidence between 20 and 30 years of age.

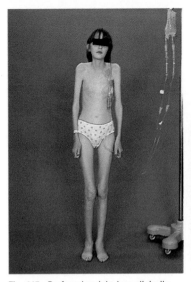

Fig. 117 Profound weight loss clinically apparent in a patient with inflammatory bowel disease. TPN had been instituted.

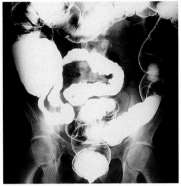

Fig. 118 Barium enema showing classical appearance of Crohn's disease of the ileum.

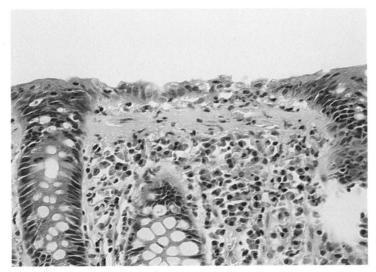

Fig. 119 Histological features of collagenous colitis.

Inflammatory bowel disease (cont.)

Aetiology   At present the aetiology of inflammatory bowel disease is unknown. Several infective agents have been proposed and an arteritis has been observed in Crohn's disease; smoking may also play a role in Crohn's disease.

Pathology   In ulcerative colitis there is inflammation limited to the mucosa without penetration of muscularis mucosa (Fig. 120) except in toxic dilatation. The inflammation and ulceration tend to be worse in the rectum and become less marked as they spread proximally along the colon. Pseudopolyps can form. In Crohn's disease the inflammation spreads through the full thickness of the bowel wall with fissures and possible fistula formation (Fig. 121). Characteristically, granulomas can be identified in Crohn's disease. Macroscopically in Crohn's disease there are patches of bowel which are relatively normal in between areas of active inflammation—so-called 'skip lesions'.

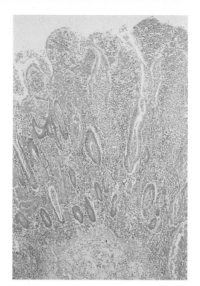

Fig. 120 Histological features of ulcerative colitis.

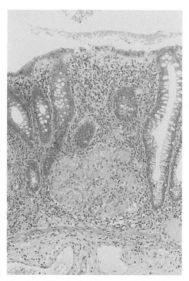

Fig. 121 Histological features of Crohn's disease.

Inflammatory bowel disease (cont.)

Complications

Gastrointestinal Crohn's disease is more commonly associated with fistula formation and fissures (Fig. 122). Toxic megacolon and perforation may occur in both forms of inflammatory bowel disease, with stricture formation more common in Crohn's disease. Colonic carcinoma is more common in patients with inflammatory bowel disease.

Occular Conjunctivitis, episcleritis and uveitis may occur in either type of inflammatory bowel disease.

Skin Erythema nodosum, pyoderma gangrenosum and oral apthous ulceration may occur.

Musculoskeletal Arthralgia, seronegative arthritides, sacroiliitis and ankylosing spondylitis (Fig. 123) can occur in inflammatory bowel disease. Ankylosing spondylitis and sacroiliitis are more common in patients with an HLA B27 phenotype.

Liver abnormalities These are multiple, including fatty change, pericholangitis, sclerosing cholangitis, amyloidosis and gallstone formation. Granulomatous hepatitis may be associated with Crohn's disease and bile duct carcinoma can complicate sclerosing cholangitis.

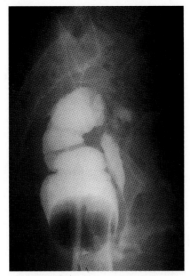

Fig. 122 Colo-vaginal fistula.

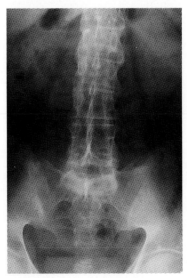

Fig. 123 Sacroiliitis and ankylosing spondylitis.

Inflammatory bowel disease (cont.)

Treatment

Diet Treatment with low residue, milk-free and elemental diets have been used in the treatment of inflammatory bowel disease.

5-ASA preparations Preparations containing 5-aminosalicylic acid may prevent relapse once the patient has attained remission (Fig. 124). There are several preparations currently available.

Steroid therapy Topical steroids can be used in rectal inflammatory bowel disease (Fig. 125). With severe acute inflammatory bowel disease (Fig. 126), intravenous or oral steroid therapy is required.

Other medical therapy Azathioprine, 6-mercaptopurine, cyclosporin A and metronidazole have all been used for the treatment of inflammatory bowel disease.

Surgical Surgery is undertaken when medical therapy has failed. It is also undertaken for patients with severe dysplasia or carcinoma of the colon. Toxic megacolon may necessitate emergency colectomy. In ulcerative colitis a total colectomy with ileostomy or ileorectal anastomosis is preferred. Crohn's disease, however, tends to recur and therefore limited resection is the operation of choice in patients with strictures or fistulae.

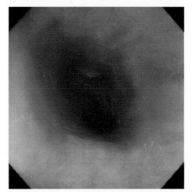

Fig. 124 Endoscopic appearance of mild inflammation and a featureless colon in a patient with ulcerative colitis.

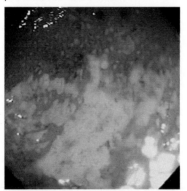

Fig. 125 Rectal ulcerative colitis.

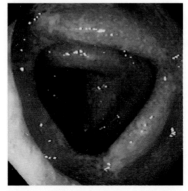

Fig. 126 Colitis affecting the transverse colon.

Diverticular disease

Definition   Herniation of the mucosa and submucosa through the muscle layer of the large bowel. Diverticulae may become inflamed and this is referred to as diverticulitis.

Clinical features   Diverticulae are often an incidental finding during colonscopic (Fig. 127) or barium enema examinations (Fig. 128). Diverticulitis is associated with systemic upset, fever and abdominal pain. Diverticular disease may also be complicated by profuse bleeding. Recurrent diverticulitis can lead to stricture formation which may be difficult to differentiate from malignancy on barium enema examination.

Treatment   Asymptomatic patients require no more than a high fibre diet. Diverticulitis is treated by antibiotics. However, diverticulitis may result in fistulae formation or general peritonitis, when surgical resection is essential. Acute haemorrhage may be treated conservatively, although surgical resection is occasionally required.

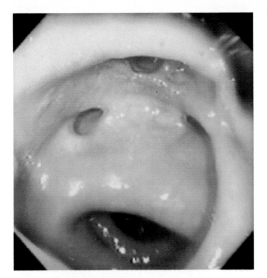

Fig. 127 Sigmoid diverticular disease.

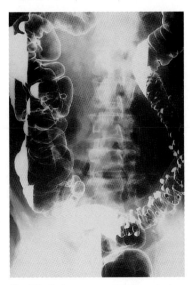

Fig. 128 Barium enema showing colonic diverticulae.

Angiodysplasia

Definition   These are arteriovenous malformations located within the colonic mucosa. They are associated with aortic valve disease, possibly through an acquired abnormality in von Willebrand's factor.

Clinical features   Angiodysplasia often causes occult gastrointestinal blood loss and may present with the symptoms of anaemia or frank rectal bleeding.

Diagnosis   The lesions may be observed at colonoscopy (Fig. 129), alternatively angiography may identify the lesion (Fig. 130).

Treatment   Diathermy or laser treatment at colonoscopy may control bleeding, however, surgical resection may be required.

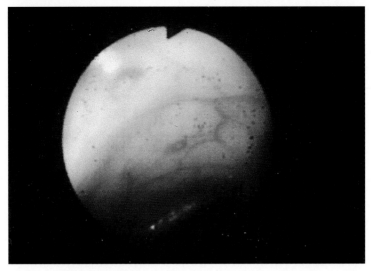

Fig. 129 Angiodysplasia identified at colonoscopy.

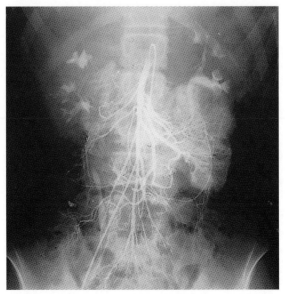

Fig. 130 Angiogram showing caecal angiodysplasia.

Ischaemic colitis

Definition Acute interruption of the blood supply affecting the large bowel with resultant necrosis.

Clinical features Abdominal pain with bloody diarrhoea and subsequent stricture formation. The location of the stricture is usually at the splenic flexure. The condition usually occurs in the elderly, but it may complicate atrial fibrillation or any other source of emboli, e.g. subacute bacterial endocarditis, or arteritis, e.g. polyarteritis nodosa. Characteristic features are found on endoscopy, biopsy and barium enema (Fig. 131).

Treatment Symptomatic treatment is sufficient in the majority of patients, but occasionally, surgical resection may be required (Fig. 132).

Radiation colitis

This usually affects the rectum and sigmoid colon following the irradiation of uterine tumours in women (Fig. 133). It presents as severe diarrhoea which is largely resistant to therapy.

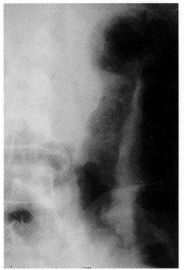

Fig. 131 Ischaemic colitis.

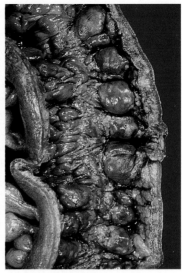

Fig. 132 Surgical resection specimen showing ischaemic colitis.

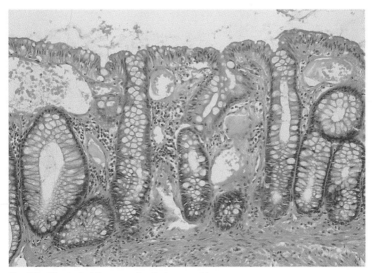

Fig. 133 Histological features of radiation proctitis.

Colonic polyps

Aetiology These may be differentiated into hyperplastic, adenomatous or villous.

Clinical features They may be a chance finding in patients being investigated for other reasons (Fig. 134), or may present with lower GI blood loss, the passage of mucous and in cases of villous adenomas, hypokalaemia due to potassium loss (Fig. 135).

Treatment Adenomatous and villous colonic polyps are premalignant and are removed endoscopically if small, although because of the risk of recurrence patients require colonoscopic surveillance (Figs 136 & 137).

Hereditary polyposis syndromes

Familial adenomatous polyposis This is an autosomally dominant condition. Multiple adenomas occur throughout the large bowel with the development of adenocarcinoma by the early twenties.

Gardner's syndrome An autosomally dominant condition in which polyps of the colon are associated with polyps throughout the bowel, mesodermal tumours and pigmented fundi.

Peutz-Jegher's syndrome This is an autosomal dominantly inherited condition in which hamartomas of the GI tract are associated with perioral buccal pigmentation. The patients may present with GI haemorrhage or intussusception. It is not a premalignant condition.

Canada-Cronkhite syndrome Metaplastic polyps of the bowel are associated with alopecia, pigmentation, nail dystrophy and malabsorption.

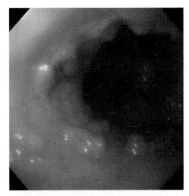

Fig. 134 Pseudopolyposis in a patient with ulcerative colitis.

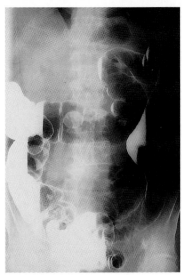

Fig. 135 Barium enema showing a colonic polyp.

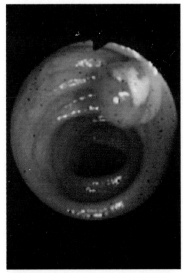

Fig. 136 Colonoscopic appearances of a sigmoid polyp.

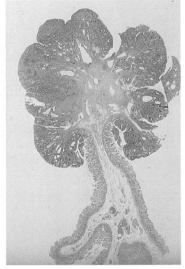

Fig. 137 Histological features of a tubular adenoma.

Colonic cancer

The most common carcinoma of the colon is adenocarcinoma. Other tumours are much less common.

Aetiology The incidence of this tumour is variable in different populations. It is more common in first degree relatives of affected patients and is increased in incidence in patients with villous, tubular or tubulovillous adenomas, ulcerative colitis and Crohn's disease, familial polyposis and Gardner's syndrome.

Clinical features A change in bowel habit with the development of constipation or diarrhoea may be the only symptom. Alternatively acute rectal bleeding or chronic occult blood loss may occur. The tumour most commonly metastasises to the liver, lung and bone which may also produce symptoms.

Diagnosis Colonoscopy or flexible sigmoidoscopy with biopsy allow the identification of tumour. A barium enema may show the presence of carcinoma (Fig. 138), but does not allow histological confirmation.

Treatment Surgical resection is undertaken if possible (Fig. 139), although radiotherapy and chemotherapy may provide benefit in patients too unfit for surgery.

Prognosis This is dependent on the degree of spread at presentation and sharply decreases if the mesenteric lymph nodes are involved with tumour.

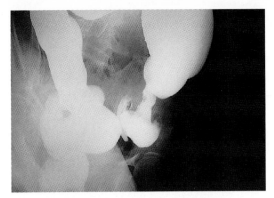

Fig. 138 Barium enema showing caecal carcinoma.

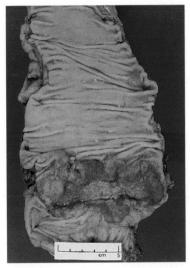

Fig. 139 Surgical resection of ulcerative rectal carcinoma with an associated polyp.

16 / **Rectum and anus**

Inflammation and infection

The rectum and anus may be involved with Crohn's disease or ulcerative colitis (Figs 139, 140, & 141). The rectal or perianal areas may be inflected with CMV or herpes viruses in immunosuppressed patients. Such patients may also develop perianal warts.

Solitary rectal ulcer syndrome

This is a benign disease which may develop secondary to prolapse of the mucosa through the anus or to self-mutilation. Patients present with diarrhoea, rectal bleeding or discomfort after opening their bowels. Diagnosis is by sigmoidoscopy and rectal biopsy. Treatment is difficult.

Haemorrhoids

This is a common condition. Haemorrhoids can be internal or external and may be complicated by haemorrhage, prolapse and strangulation or mucous discharge with perianal itching. Treatment is dependent upon the degree of the piles, but may simply require laxatives. Alternatively, injection, rubber band ligation or surgical resection may be required.

Fissure in-ano

This is a split in the anal mucosa usually occurring posteriorly secondary to increased straining. It presents with pain on defaecation and haemorrhage and is treated with stool softeners or anal dilators.

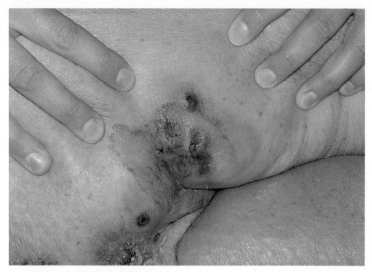

Fig. 140 Perianal Crohn's disease.

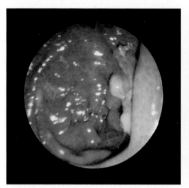

Fig. 141 Melanosis coli following laxative abuse.

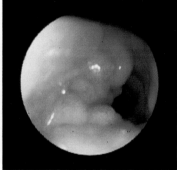

Fig. 142 Pneumatosis coli.

Index